SCOTT LEWIS

Staying Safe for Today's Woman

Recognize and Avoid Predators

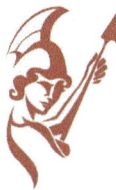

ATHENA WOMEN
CONFIDENT AWARENESS

This book is dedicated to my wife and life partner, Gail,
and to our adult children Kevin and Erica.
Their assistance and support throughout the many hours I've spent training and
teaching made this book and training possible.

"Awareness will save you more than any technique I could ever show."

Guro Ron Balicki, Martial Arts Research Systems

Contents

Preface

STAYING SAFE FOR TODAY'S WOMAN
The Awareness And Avoidance Strategies Of
Athena Women Self-Protection Training

For People With Long-term, Short-term, or No Training

I understand feeling small and overpowered.

The average American adult male outweighs me by over 30 pounds and is also usually stronger than I am. But being small doesn't have to mean feeling out of control or lacking confidence. It does, however, call for being aware, thinking ahead, and understanding predators. **This book is all about training your brain to intentionally stay one step ahead of predators.**

A big step toward confidence and a sense of control: Some of our Athena Women Self Protection students have told us they notice, recognize, and avoid questionable persons that they would not have identified before training with us.

While this book does serve as a reference for Athena Women Self Protection training, I planned and wrote *Staying Safe for Today's Woman* to also be stand-alone useful to the vast majority of you who cannot attend our—or perhaps any—training. As with our physical training, this book focuses on awareness skills, improving your understanding of victim and predator habits, recognizing and avoiding threatening people and situations, and verbal and physical de-escalation techniques.

Predators use our physiology and habits against us. You will refine how you stay ahead of predators to beat them at their own game. To aid you in that, this book gives you practice with some of the non-contact scenarios we use in our training. Women with awareness-focused training are much less likely to be targeted for assault.

Practicing awareness and avoidance skills is required to make them a habit, but takes no time. Do them during your normal routines.

If you've survived an attack, kudos for summoning the courage to open this book to help you regain confidence and improve your control over your safety.

While this book does not attempt to instruct you in fighting skills, *the head work skills you will learn in this book are <u>the most important</u> advantage of Athena Women Self Protection classes.*

This book may lead you to seek training in self protection that includes fighting skills. For ideas about that decision, please refer to the Training Tips chapter.

Acknowledgement

After I was medically grounded from airline piloting, my wife and partner Gail suggested I create a short-term women's self-defense course as a new endeavor, and she helped screen techniques. My law enforcement officer son Kevin (who, in addition to his police training studied at Kreimer's Karate, wrestled and has trained in Brazilian Jiu Jitsu; his ground fighting skills far exceed mine) and my daughter Erica also assisted in the selection and refinement of Athena Women techniques. We all owe them thanks.

This course would not be possible without the rigorous training I received at Kreimer's Karate Institute. Thank you to Grandmaster Ralph F. Kreimer, Manager and Instructor Linda Kreimer, and Chief Instructor Adam Kreimer for their encouragement to develop this course.

The list of coaches and teammates as well as fellow students and instructors who helped and encouraged me over the decades is long. It includes my wrestling coaches and teammates, instructors in judo and Shotokan karate I dabbled in while young, and the many high-quality instructors and students I've had the privilege of training and competing with at Kreimer's Karate Institute and other schools around the US.

Thanks also to this course's students. I appreciate their enthusiasm and always candid input. They helped make this training more efficient and user-friendly.

Westview Psychological Counseling Service answered questions I had about predators and victims. (WPCS did not have input into the mental illness discussion herein.)

During the 1998 running of "Karate College" at Radford University, I attended workshops by undefeated former PKA world champion Bill "Superfoot" Wallace. Later I mentioned to Grandmaster Wallace that I'd recently read his book, *Dynamic Stretching and Kicking.* He encouraged me to write my own book about martial arts.

To the many airline coworkers and other friends who urged me to "write your book," thank you.

Special thanks go to generous members of the law enforcement community (including my son) who were crucial in guiding me in the selection of topics in this book, and their critique of corresponding areas of training in the Athena Women course. Their help and spirit were vital to this effort. I back the blue.

Scott Lewis

November, 2023

1

BREAK THE ERROR CHAIN

"When I first started coaching, one of the worst things that I think I heard was 'It will be O.K.' I would wonder, 'How...is it going to be O.K.?' The worst word in the English language is 'hope.'" — *Coach Bobby Knight*

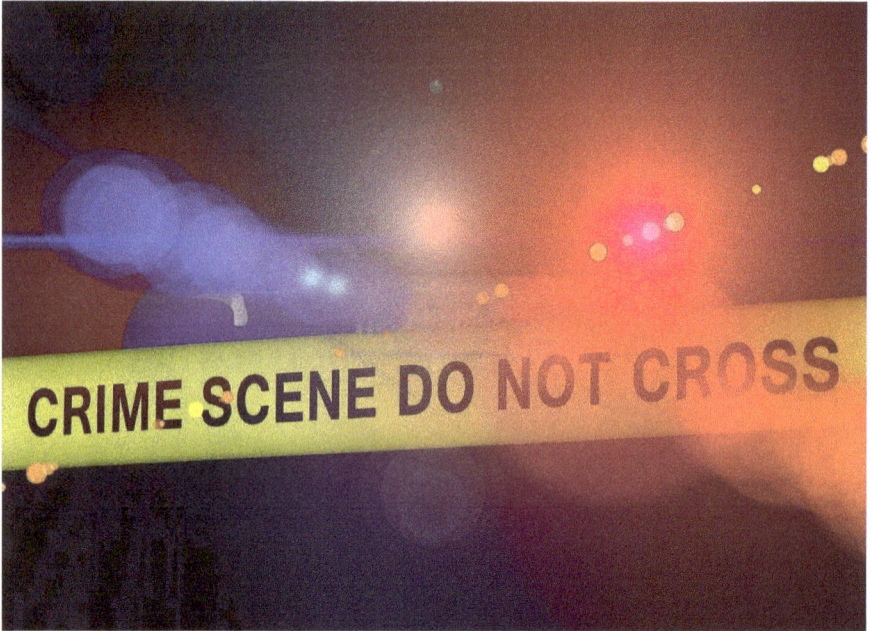

Our goal is to help you to never be inside this tape.

You look idly around the theater lobby then open your purse and glance at the time on your phone. One o'clock in the morning already? You'd rather have attended the earlier showing but you had to work late. You got the text about the late movie from your night owl friends who never seem to make plans until after most people are asleep. By now you're used to it. You caved. *Sure, let's see a movie.* So you texted your family before you left, but there was no reply. They were sleeping, along with the rest of the world. No wonder they let you use the car. So you picked up your friends and drove to the movie, and now you have to drop them off.

Your two friends are stepping out of the rest room. You feel as if you're in a different time zone, that time has skipped a little ahead of you. What was a bustling, noisy room just moments ago is now eerily hushed and almost empty, save for you three, a couple holding hands, and a guy in a mall uniform who just passed through the lobby and slipped into a back room. You notice you are now invisible to the workers cleaning up—the same ones who eagerly assisted you two hours ago. Somehow, a public place designed to welcome a large crowd feels harsh and uninviting when empty. Time to leave, you and the other stragglers. Friends in tow, you push open the door and feel the cold breeze on your face. You just want to be in the warm car, on your way home.

Even at eleven o'clock, you had to park what seemed like a soccer field from the building's entrance. Now the nearly deserted parking lot means you can already see the vehicle you drove here, but somehow it looks even further away.

The only thing more unsettling than being sure you're alone somewhere is *not* knowing whether you are alone. You can't stop looking around the parking lot, which should be empty but isn't quite. *Something's not quite right.*

A chill of wind and all three of you pick up your pace a little. Unlit signs tell you that you're no longer welcome in the now-darkened landscape with locked stores and closed restaurants. You detour around a small SUV as you step off the sidewalk onto the lot's pavement and angle to the right, toward your waiting car. You love the freedom that the car represents, not having to depend on your parents to chauffeur you and your friends. But it also occurs to you that if you were being picked up, the three of you would now be getting into someone's parents' warm vehicle and you'd be on your way to a comfy bed.

Despite your fatigue, you try to play along with your friends' conversation about the movie. Sure, you'd have come up with a less predictable ending, but your mind is on getting to the car—you're halfway there now. As your friends chatter, you glance up and really see the car—and two close-by parked cars—for the first time. Around them are about a half-dozen men, talking. Loudly. You don't recall seeing them in the theater. The only other nearby businesses still open are a fast food joint and a bar. The cars are closer to the latter. These boisterous men have been drinking and plan to drive.

Maybe they won't notice us.

Your friends don't seem to notice them. You are the only one worrying, so you're probably overreacting. Calm down. You're in a group, like you've been taught. Now just a few more rows to cross and you'll be fine. You don't really hear or track your friends' conversation anymore. Your friends laugh at something and one of the men notices your group for the first time. He doesn't look away.

Staring straight into you, he says something to his cohorts, and they immediately fall silent. Five other faces turn to observe your "safety" group, which is suddenly ridiculously small and insignificant. The edges of the parking lot seem to stretch to the horizon. You feel like exposed prey on the open savanna, and something is rustling in the bushes.

Your friends finally notice the men. You're walking at the same speed but for some reason your progress toward the car is never ending. You start fishing in your purse for your key fob but of course it has settled to the bottom. Your hand movements quicken. You can't decide where to look—at the car, the men, or for the fob. So your eyes bounce between them, too fast for your brain to register. Your throat tightens a little. You become aware of your heart racing.

More talk within the group of young men while your friends have become quiet. Should you be talking, pretending to ignore them? Making sure they know you see them? *Why is it taking so long to get to the stupid car?*

Your vehicle is now about halfway between you and those men. One of them calls out to you, more loudly than needed. Then he begins to shuffle your way. The rest of his group follows. He's evidently their leader, and he's leading them to you. Now you can see that they are older than you by several years, so they can see you are much younger. *Why are they still walking toward us?*

They will get to your car before you do. In your purse, your hand now scrapes the bottom for the unlocking fob.

You break free of your anxiety for a moment and finally look around. Behind you, even. A few cold, dark, empty cars—no other people. Then you remember you walked past the shopping plaza's security SUV as you stepped off the sidewalk. It's always parked there, right in front, as much a part of the scenery as a tree. It's still there, but unoccupied. You wonder where the guard is. It now occurs to you he was the guy who walked through the lobby, but you didn't pay attention to him. An unused player in your real-life video game.

You look ahead. Two of the other men are now saying some things addressed to you. Where have you been? It's still early, where are you going? Do you want to go to our house and party? Phrased as questions, but they sound like demands. You are nearing your car from the passenger side, but the men walk around both bumpers and trap you in. On purpose?

You know you shouldn't keep walking toward the car, yet if you make a break for the theater, they will get to you before you reach it. The fast-food place is beyond the men, as is the bar. Your two escape routes have closed.

The men stop, a couple of them leaning against your mom's car. The cold wind carries the smell of stale alcohol. You still haven't found the fob, but now you are holding your cellphone. Too late, your priority has shifted from driving to survival. You realize they can get to you faster than you can dial. You might get 9-1-1 punched in, but there are no police cars in sight. As if by order, the three of you stop at once, a couple of car lengths from your vehicle and the men. You're afraid to look at them, afraid to not look at them. The men who are leaning on the car, apparently sensing your indecision, stand up, alert, like leopards picking up the scent of prey. All six are looking in your direction. Silence.

For the first time in your life you know you are helpless, and you don't know what to do.

"We made too many wrong mistakes." —Yogi Berra

What could the young women at the theater have done differently?

- Waited for a different night on which all of them could have gone to an earlier showing. Was going that particular night important enough to accept the risk of the later hour? **Acting for your safety can be inconvenient.**
- **Planned ahead** regarding the movie ending so late, and not parked close to a bar since some of its patrons would be well-oiled by the end of the movie.
- *Noticed* (paid attention) that the man in the mall uniform was the security guard; they could have asked him to walk or drive them to their car. He was an unused resource.

5

- When they walked past the mall security SUV, they could have turned around, re-entered the theater and asked for the guard—or called someone's parents and waited inside. Willingness to adjust to changing circumstances can save your life.
- Stopped. Made a decision to change course when they first felt uneasy about activity in the parking lot. **Always honor the gut feeling that tells you something is *not* right.** That's your personal radar. More about that ahead.
- They could have kept their heads on swivels to spot trouble sooner. We give you an orderly way to do this.
- They didn't plan, keep track of escape routes, or notice their options were disappearing as they got closer to their car, which left them no way out. More on escape routes later, too.
- As soon as one of them spotted the crowd around their car, they should have made the immediate decision to turn around or detour widely to the fast-food restaurant (avoid), and wait for the drunks to leave the scene or call for help. They *hoped* the men wouldn't notice them. **If you catch yourself thinking "I hope..." that's a Red Flag (a warning that your plan is falling apart).**
- One of the young women began worrying, but she let the fact that her friends seemed unconcerned influence her decision. That's called *herding*, and it can be dangerous. **She should have listened to her gut—and acted on that feeling.**

2

ATHENA WOMEN PHILOSOPHY

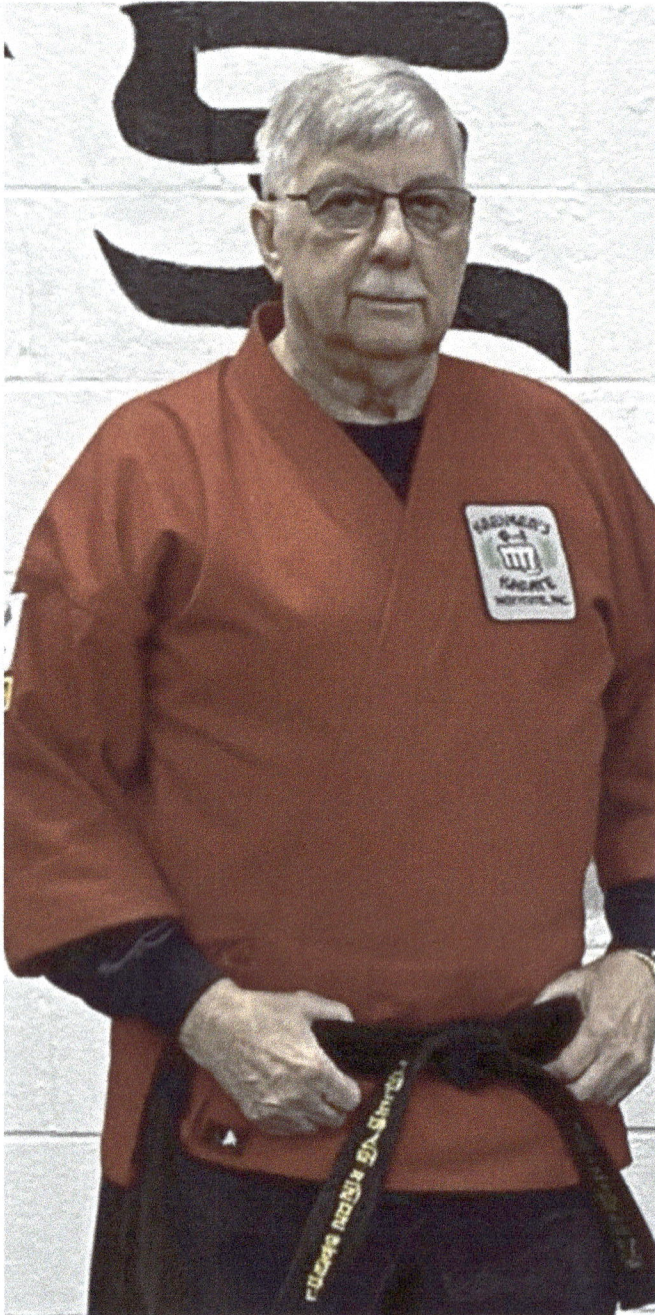

"You can do anything if you are patient, take your time and work hard. No time is wasted." —My Sensei, 9th Dan Grandmaster Ralph F. Kreimer

W elcome to life-changing information.

This book teaches self-*protection*, which is taking initiative to stay safe by avoiding predators and physical confrontations that would require self-defense fighting skills. *Staying Safe for Today's Woman* presents the awareness and avoidance tactics from our Athena Women Self-Protection training. Our awareness-first approach works: To the best of our knowledge, none of our in-class graduates have had to physically fight an attacker. That's our mission. Train with us or read this book and you will learn about common assault venues, predators, and how to recognize and avoid them. You'll also learn about yourself—about the vulnerabilities that we all share and which predators use against us.

As a long-time fighting arts instructor, retired flight instructor and airline pilot, I believe that self-protection training benefits from current pilot training methods. Our whole-cloth method of teaching responses from the very beginning of evolving, chaotic, dynamic assault scenarios is a page taken from modern pilot training. The outcome of each situation is influenced by the you choices you make, among other factors. Like real life.

Old-school flight training relied on teaching canned responses to tightly scripted, catastrophic emergencies. The newer, more reality-oriented approach is designed to train pilots to respond to complex, evolving, unpredictable situations requiring nuanced judgment using all available resources—exactly the thinking that can also keep you safe in a parking garage after dark.

To the untrained, an assault may seem to start with close, sudden violence, requiring little decision-making and a fight-for-your-life reaction (old school training). A trained person would recognize that the very same event actually started earlier as the assailant lured his victim into distracting dialogue. You will recognize and be wary of such predator tactics after reading this book (modern reality-based training). Using the awareness, verbal, and de-escalating responses you'll learn, you might escape a threatening situation without needing to physically fight. For examples of common attack situations, in the Pulling It All Together chapter, I've detailed some awareness and avoidance training scenarios that we teach in our classes for you to practice (these drills do not involve any physical contact between the participants).

The following warnings probably confirm your suspicions:

- **Violent attacks are brutal, chaotic, and *overwhelming*. There are no rules.**
- **During an attack you will not have the time or space you want to fight back, his attack will injure you more than you're prepared for, and your strikes will be less effective than you hoped. An attack on you can result in serious or fatal injury.**
- **Do not physically engage a Threat unless there is no other choice (more on this ahead). This is even more crucial if the Threat is armed.**

Given the above, clearly awareness and avoidance are the foundation of self-protection. We offer simple ways to stay aware of your environment and identify and avoid threats. We show you how to set boundaries (your "bubble"). These skills can help you discern whether an approaching person has intent to do you harm, so you can be confident (tactically and legally) in your decision to avoid, de-escalate, flee, give up your valuables, or as a last resort prepare to fight.

Predators want victims, not fights.

Women trained in *modern awareness-based* self-protection project awareness and confidence and therefore are far less often targeted for attack.[1] This reflects the fact that animal and human predators target those that appear to be the easiest prey. If you have to choose between either short-term training in awareness skills or short-term training in fighting skills, choose awareness skills first.

Most victims of sexual assault know their attackers.[2] Rather than assuming

---

[1] "Success Rate of Graduates Fighting Back—Stopping Violence Against Women" (accessed April 20, 2021); available from http://modelmugging.org/success-rate-of-graduates-fighting-back/

[2] "Perpetrators of Sexual Violence: Statistics" (accessed December 20, 2017); available from https://www.rainn.org/statistics/perpetrators-sexual-violence

you can predict what other people's brains will decide to do in the future[3], use the strategies you will learn in this book to **avoid providing opportunities for stealth predators to attack you.**

Our training is named after the Greek mythological figure Athena. Greek myth holds that she was recognized primarily for her wisdom, but when she had to fight, she did so ferociously.

Welcome to life-changing knowledge.

* * *

Because online self-protection videos routinely disappear, many videos I would recommend will be deleted by the time you read this. However, news stations tend to leave their videos up. Television station WDVM ran a story about our Athena Women Self Protection training. Click HERE[4] for the two-minute video. Note: the violent crime (murder, rape, robbery, aggravated assault) statistic I quote in the video is for the city of Frederick, MD, the home of our training.

THIS[5] is a good introduction to self-protection training by a Krav Maga school.

Note both schools' emphasis on awareness.

---

[3] "Prediction is very difficult, especially if it's about the future". —physicist **Niels Bohr**

[4] "Local Studio is Teaching Women How To Punch, Kick and Stomp" (accessed November 10, 2023); available from https://www.dcnewsnow.com/news/local-studio-is-teaching-women-how-to-punch-kick-and-stomp/

[5] "Free Women's Safety Training This Week" (accessed November 10, 2023); available from https://rumble.com/v8xtqf-free-womens-safety-training-this-week.html

3

LEGALLY SPEAKING

hether in this book or in our classes, we always advocate you avoid violence and if that is not possible, you use only justifiable force. The discussion below is only a rough sketch of the very, very complex issue of justifiable use of force in the United States.

Consult an attorney: *Once you use force, you enter the Byzantine criminal justice system and you do not control the outcome.*

- Essentially, assault is an attempted or actual unwanted, harmful, or offensive touch.
- You don't have to be injured to call the police.

Using force against another person is against the law. If you use force, even in your defense, you are violating the law. When you violate the law, it becomes *up to you to prove* that your violation was justified.* This is another reason for steering clear of violence by honing awareness and avoidance skills including those presented in this book. Becoming more knowledgeable about predators and self-defense can keep you out of jail as well as out of the ER.

*In order for fighting back to be judged as justifiable use of force:

- You are not the attacker and do not start the fight.
- You must have a *reasonable basis* to believe you are in *imminent* danger

of being *injured*. Reasonable basis: the person has the opportunity, capability and *intent* to harm you. Imminent means the injury *will occur now unless someone intervenes*.

· You have to *actually believe* you are in *imminent* danger of being *injured*.
· You do not use more than a *reasonable* amount of force to repel the attack unless it is necessary to use deadly force (e.g., you fear for your life).
· In some circumstances you must have no other option (such as fleeing).
· Justifiable use of force ends when the danger has passed.

Simplifying that checklist, according to police the use of force can be deemed justifiable if you are being physically assaulted or are being <u>physically *(not merely verbally)* threatened with a physical assault</u>, so long as you use the appropriate level of force only until the danger has passed. Reread those bullet points and notice nowhere do they state you have to passively allow a 250 pound thug to knock you in the head, likely ending the "fight," before you use force to protect yourself. (Intent is key—more on that ahead.)

The outcome of a self-defense case depends on the crime location's statutes and case law, and the associated judgments of the investigating officer, prosecuting attorney, as well as judge and jury if the case goes to trial. In addition to understanding the law, you should be aware of how self-defense laws are interpreted and applied in the jurisdiction of the event—before you use force.

For a non-attorney's discussion of what self-defense is see HERE [6] and about the legal aftermath see HERE [7]

Know your location's laws with respect to self-defense, castle doctrine,

---

[6] "No Nonsense Self-Defense" (accessed November 10, 2023); available from http://nononsen seselfdefense.com/self-defenseexplained.htm

[7] "No Nonsense Self-Defense (Legal Aftermath) (accessed November 10, 2023); available from "http://nononsenseselfdefense.com/legal.html

stand your ground and duty to retreat HERE [8], HERE [9]. (Reference Maryland's self-defense laws HERE.[10])

Each self-defense case will be judged based on five elements: innocence, imminence, reasonableness, avoidance and proportionality. HERE [11]

---

[8] "Self Defense (United States)" (accessed September 29, 2023); available from https://encyclopedia.thefreedictionary.com/Self-defense+(United+States)

[9] "Stand Your Ground (35 States) vs. Duty to Retreat (15 States)" (accessed September 29, 2023); available from https://reason.com/volokh/2020/12/21/duty-to-retreat-35-states-vs-stand-your-ground-15-states/

[10] "Maryland self-defense laws" (accessed November 10, 2023); available from https://www.findlaw.com/state/maryland-law/maryland-self-defense-laws.html

[11] "Self-Defense Law: The 5 Elements for Justified Use of Force" (accessed September 29, 2023); available from https://www.arsenalattorneys.com/firearms-blog/self-defense-case-study-frank-trujillo

4

THE ATHENA WOMEN FIVE STEP PLAN

"It's about you being one step ahead of your attacker. That's the most important thing; I can't stress it enough." —Nick Drossos of **Code Red Defense**™ [12]

---

[12] "Most Important Part of Self Defense" (accessed April 28, 2018); available from https://www.youtube.com/watch?v=AsRd1uVW3cM

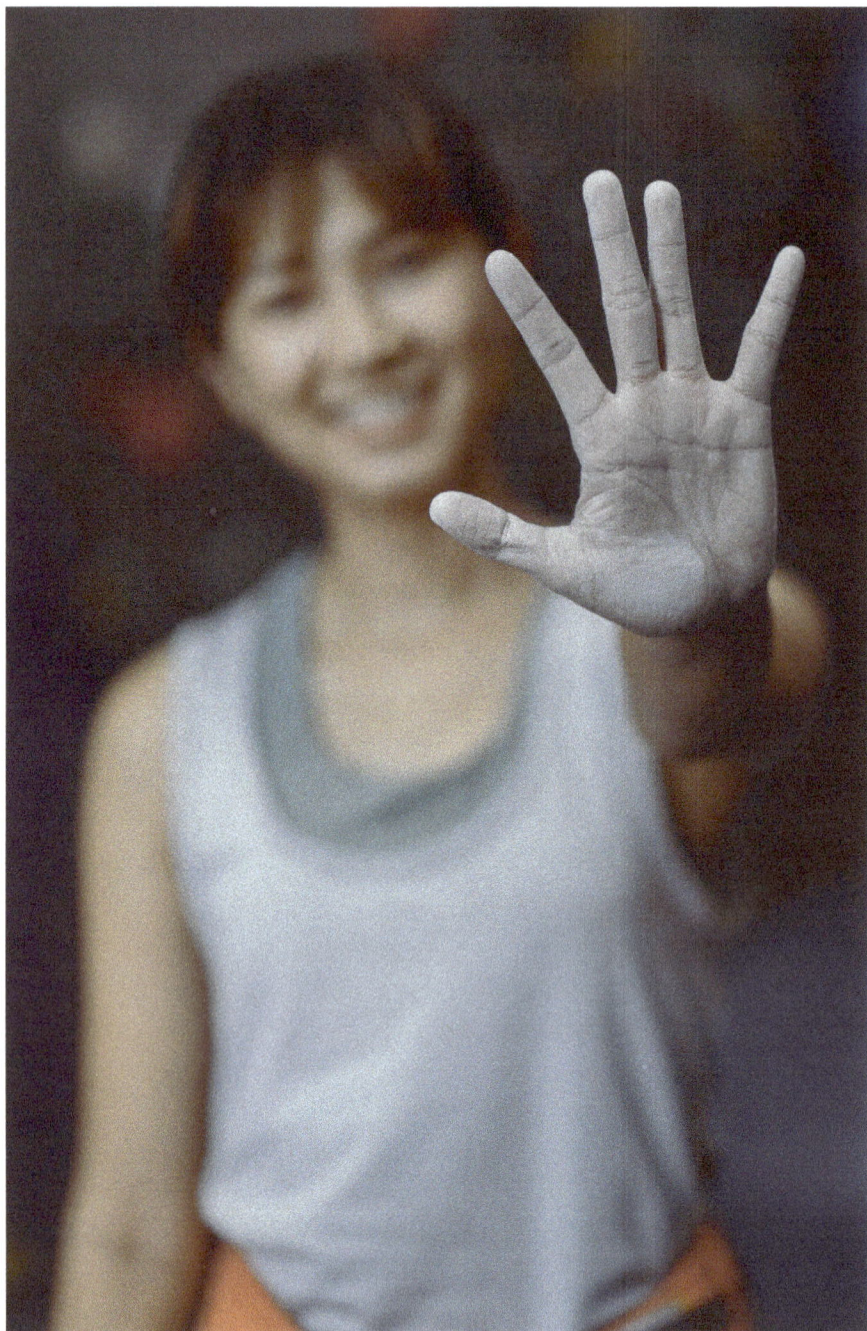

Photo: Allan Mas

T he Athena Women **Five Step Plan**:

Aware

Includes recognizing threats; keep your head on a swivel (we have an organized method)

Avoid/Deescalate

Try to always have two safe places to move to when necessary. Deescalation is an avoidance tool.

Flee

Running away beats fighting any day. Anytime during a confrontation that fleeing *safely* (e.g., you won't be attacked from behind) becomes an option, take it.

Comply

If you're unable to flee safely, complying may include walking away, turning over your valuables as the assailant demands before he's close enough to touch you, or not taking an opportunity to argue. *Complying does* **not** *imply yielding to a sexual attack and* **never** *includes allowing the predator to relocate you to the "second crime scene."* Among other atrocities, the second crime scene is where the body is found. Allowing a predator to take you to another location is *not* safely complying. If safely complying doesn't stop the thug from attacking you...

(Counter)Attack

In all cases when we say "attack" we mean **justifiable** *counterattack using* **reasonable force** *in response to the* **physical** *actions of a Threat* **until the danger has passed**.

You absolutely must get very proficient at those first four steps so that you never get to step five—especially if you lack the opportunity to train in fighting back.

Victims frequently express shock and incredulity at the degree of evil, sadistic cruelty attackers needlessly dispense. A predator can inflict disabling and serious injury with a single punch.

Naturally, our Five Step Plan is a neat, clean theory for a messy reality. Fleeing safely may not be possible if the attacker sneaked up on you or if you think he can, and will, run faster to catch you if you flee. Paying attention to your environment can provide you with the opportunity to escape before you are approached by a questionable individual or provide you with the opportunity of tossing your valuables before a robber is close enough to do you harm, perhaps giving you time to flee while he collects your valuables. Practicing scenarios yields huge improvement in your judgment and confidence.

Our Training Works

Our students have told us that they notice people around them that they wouldn't have spared a second glance prior to training with us. One student spotted a man stalking her during her run in a city park and was able to flee while he was still distant enough for her to safely outrun him.

The Pulling It All Together chapter discusses in detail implementing the Five Step Plan.

What "Captain Sully" and F/O Stiles Teach Us About Survival

Let's look at an incident you are aware of that a movie later called a "miracle". To refresh your memory, on January 15, 2009, Captain Chesley "Sully" Sullenberger and First Officer Jeff Skiles flying USAirways Flight 1549 made a remarkable decision under pressure and saved 155 lives. After suffering numerous bird strikes, including to both engines, from a flock of geese just three minutes after takeoff from New York's LaGuardia airport, the twin-engine Airbus 321 they were flying suffered an extremely rare dual engine failure. Air traffic controllers cleared the airspace and runways at nearby airports but the crew informed them that the airplane never reached sufficient altitude to be able to glide (unpowered) to land at any of the nearby airports. A mere four minutes after takeoff Captain Sully told ATC, "We're gonna be in the Hudson."[13] A ditching, sometimes euphemistically called a "water landing", was their decision.

The pilots displayed professionalism and sharp skills, yet in my view the real miracle was the crew's *fast recognition* of the threat, *correct analysis of their rapidly worsening flight condition* and *bold decision—skills needed to stay safe on the ground as well.* For you non-pilots, consider: these two pilots had made tens of thousands of landings—one per takeoff—for their entire careers. Putting an airline jet with 155 people on board into a river only a few minutes after a routine takeoff defines the cliché "nerves of steel" (they avoided falling prey to expectation bias—see the Challengers & Tools chapter.)

These individuals had the mindset to do whatever was necessary to survive. As with a self-protection situation, it was their *awareness* and *decision making* that put them in a position to make the best of their survival skills. Poor awareness or decision making—or delayed decision making—would have put them in a position that no degree of skill could have made survivable. How do we develop the *pilot's proactive survival mindset*?

The same way pilots do: through repeatedly thinking through "what if" scenarios.

As with facing a predator:

- Their day had been unremarkable, with no signs of an imminent threat.
- Everything went well until a sudden, unpredictable crisis erupted.
- The decision they were called on to make would save or kill them (and 153 others).
- They had seconds to make that decision, which would be irreversible. No do-over.

---

[13] "Hero pilot 'Sully' Sullenberger recalls 'Miracle on the Hudson' landing 10 years later" (accessed January 14, 2020); available from https://www.nydailynews.com/new-york/ny-metro-hudson-miracle-landing-20190114-story.html

· Victims vacillate; defenders decide.

Can I Really Do This?

The confidence and resulting lowered stress that you take away from aware-ness or fighting training spills over to all areas of life. Once you **realize** that not "everyone is just like me" and some of them are scary and want to do you harm, and you **internalize the mindset** to be on the lookout for and proactively **deal with evil on your terms**, that is a life-changing realization and mindset you cannot undo. Congratulations.

Confidence

"All martial artists are beginners; some of us have just been beginning a little longer!"
   —Hapkido Grandmaster J. R. West[14]

Fortunately, confidence doesn't require certainty that you can prevail in any violent confrontation. No one is granted that guarantee. ***Confidence is the assurance of knowing you can execute your self protection plan because you've practiced it many times.*** A lack of confidence is distracting and distractions can kill.

* * *

"Sensei Ando" gives REALISTIC, UPBEAT ADVICE[15] about being prepared without being paranoid. From the video: "When you make safety a habit, you

---

[14] "West's Hapkido" (accessed January 3, 2020); available from https://hapkido.com

[15] "Self-Defense Against a Sucker Punch" (accessed November 10, 2023); available from https://www.youtube.com/watch?v=qJLdXitWlaI

don't have to worry about it anymore."

A sucker punch is a common beginning to some violent crimes, and Sensei Ando is correct that it's virtually impossible to evade or protect yourself from it once it's on its way toward you. In addition to his advice, you *can* train to recognize when someone is *about to* throw a sucker punch—and what to do about it.

5

YOUR CHALLENGES & TOOLS

"**A** true martial artist embodies two traits: alertness in situations of calm; and composure in situations of chaos." — Carlos Alejandrino[16]

---

[16] Carlos Alejandrino, "Martial artist tangles with 2 road-raging attackers at once" http://www. mixedmartialarts.com/vault/street/martial-artist-tangles-with-2-road-raging-attackers -at-once, accessed June 28, 2017

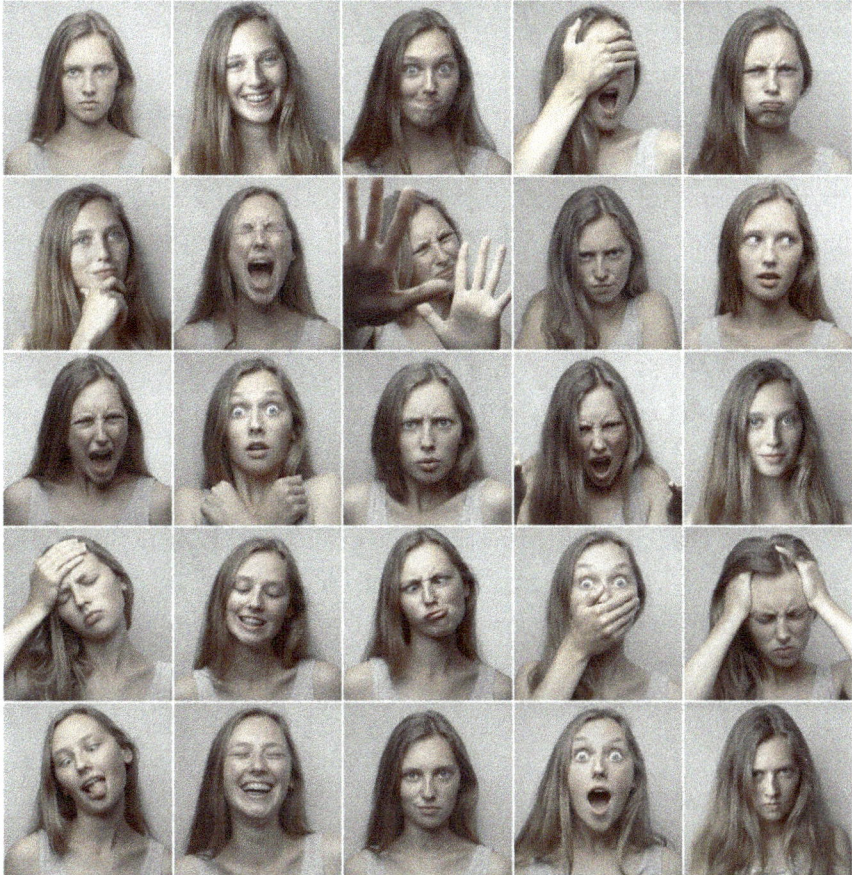

Photo: Andrea Piacquadio

What You Can Learn From Fighting Training Even If You Don't Learn To Fight

Not wanting to fight is a healthy instinct of course. Most predators don't want fights; they want *victims*, and they plan to use every advantage they can to take what they want from you. This section discusses some human vulnerabilities predators take advantage of.

It is now well-known that even soldiers in combat sometimes intentionally miss when shooting at enemies. Most of us refuse to hurt others—even to the point of being hurt ourselves; even our survival instinct can stop short of

23

harming other humans.

Years ago I was in a discussion with a group of men and women when the subject of personal security arose. One individual clung to his prideful "nonviolent" rule of refusing to strike anyone for any reason to the point that when I presented a scenario of a violent attack on him and his wife, he stubbornly refused to say he'd fight against the attacker who was beating and injuring her. This is planned—and sickening—cowardice.

Standing around with his hands in his pockets uttering pleas while his wife is getting beaten is clearly anything but nonviolent (his wife wasn't present to comment on his passivity). He evidently believed that his wife getting seriously injured was morally superior to him striking the thug. His wedding vows—*love, honor and cherish*—must have slipped his mind. When violence is underway, the nonviolence option has already fled the scene. That is the attacker's doing. We adults know that we can only play the cards we are dealt.

If you're opposed to all violence, to be consistent you must be opposed to violence to everyone—not everyone *except* you (or a family member). If you refuse to fight back, your decision will probably increase the total violence done. Your attacker will hurt you more than you would hurt him because you are required to use only reasonable force. He doesn't operate under a civilized rule of doing minimum harm.

The surest way to halt the violence is to stop the attacker. *You are worth fighting for.* If you need more authoritative reassurance, look up 1 Samuel 21:8, Matthew 12:29, Luke 11:21 and 22:36.

How Predators Use Your Physiology Against You

Now, onto how your mind and body will *involuntarily* react during a violent assault.

"...high-level SNS [Sympathetic Nervous System] activation occurs when combatants are confronted with an unanticipated deadly force threat and the time to respond is minimal. Under these conditions the extreme effects of the SNS will cause catastrophic failure of the visual, cognitive, and motor control systems. Although there are endless variables that may trigger the

SNS, there are six key variables that have an immediate impact of the level of SNS activation. These are: the degree of malevolent, human intent behind the threat; the perceived level of threat, ranging from risk of injury to the potential for death; the time available to response [sic]; *the level of* **confidence** *in personal skills and training; the level of* **experience** *in dealing with the specific threat; and the degree of physical fatigue that is combined with the anxiety.*" [Emphasis added][17]

You can control the last three factors and possibly the time available if you're alert. Give yourself more time to respond by having 360-degree awareness through proper attention to your environment and not waiting "to see what happens." Increase your confidence by having good training habits. Raise your experience through ongoing training in many scenarios and mentally working through what you would do in an assault (see the Pulling It All Together chapter). Reduce physical fatigue by exercising enough to stay in shape. In training to meet violence, you might reduce how much the "fog of war" affects your ability to see, hear, think, and act.

Athena Women training uses selected techniques based on guidelines that consider the physiological effects of a violent confrontation. Our methods are easy to remember and perform using gross motor movements, which are effective against bigger and stronger attackers and usable by average women with no prior training. Apply those standards to any training you enroll in.

Those Six Factors In Action: A Tale Of Two Confrontations

A dumb predator and a trained defender with a plan and time to execute it:

On a sunny day in a business district, a martial arts instructor looks out the window of his second story studio and sees two adult males approach another adult male across the street. No other pedestrians are in sight. One of the two hangs back several feet while the other moves in closer to the intended victim. The would-be assailant's body language indicates he is ramping up to attack:

---

[17] "Psychological Effects of Combat" (accessed February 17, 2017); available from https://www. killology.com/psychological-effects-of-combat

as he speaks, the attacker's shoulders square up, chest puffs out, head tilts forward, and his arms stiffen.

The instructor's protector mindset kicks in and he runs downstairs to the aid of the intended victim. He interposes himself between the victim-to-be and the main assailant. Determined to get to his intended victim and not bothering assess the changed situation, the perpetrator tries to attack the instructor, who knocks out the bad guy with a single punch. The attacker's accomplice, evidently the wiser of the two, keeps a safe distance from the instructor.

In this incident, the martial artist appeared to control four of those six factors that affect our SNS activation: he had *available time* to surveil the situation. He clearly had *confidence* in his skill set, likely arisen from *experience* drilling this scenario, and he *wasn't fatigued by anxiety.*

Let's list the uncommon advantages this situation conveyed to the instructor (the assailant's newly intended victim):

1. Crucially, the instructor volunteered to be involved in this situation and could have withdrawn at any time.
2. The attack took place during daylight hours.
3. The attack developed slowly.
4. The instructor observed the entire situation from a distance, knew the number of assailants and could verify their hands were empty.
5. He had time to make a rational decision using his full cognitive skills.
6. He had confidence borne of countless sparring rounds that he could fight effectively. He trusted his training and practice.
7. Once engaging the threat, the instructor had the trained advantage of recognizing an imminent assault and his movements were as quick as a startle reaction because of hundreds of thousands of practice repetitions.

An experienced predator with a plan and an untrained, time-compressed defender:

Athena Women was training this situation since before this incident occurred. An attack on a young woman outside a round-the-clock health club at night was recorded on a "security" video camera[18] and ended very badly for the victim.

A woman walked out of the club into the nearly empty parking lot. As she approached a small group of cars a man exited his vehicle and began walking toward the club. He wore sunglasses and was not carrying anything into the club. The woman and the man walked in opposite directions, separated by one column of cars. Neither of them appeared to pay any attention to the other. As they passed, the attacker made a U-turn around the vehicle separating them, which put him immediately behind her. He approached her from behind and attacked her with a haymaker punch to the side of her head, then grabbed and restrained her. He took her to the ground face-down and began to beat her. The video I saw ended there but reportedly he struck her 39 times—and he was a large, young individual. Thirty-nine punches to someone who could not defend herself means her injuries were serious—if not life threatening—and changed her life forever in a number of ways.

What about those six factors that affect our ability to react? It seems most were working against her, virtually shutting down any ability to act in defense:

1. High degree of malevolent intent
2. High level of threat of harm
3. No time to respond because she didn't maintain 360 awareness
4. She appeared to be untrained in fighting—not because she couldn't fight off someone bigger who surprised her from behind, but because she did not maintain awareness
5. A non-fighter would not likely be confident in fighting skills
6. She had no time to be fatigued from anxiety, but was possibly drained

---

[18] The predator wore sunglasses as a counter to the video camera. So much for the "security" it provided the savagely beaten victim. Security cameras should be considered "evidence cameras".

from exercising

We train "different is a **Red Flag**" (a seemingly small detail pointing to a larger problem). When watching people, you instinctively know to look out for those behaving oddly. Let's count the **Red Flags** and examine how well this attack was engineered and executed:

1. The man hopped out of his car just as the woman was approaching. What convenient timing. What are the chances that late at night, with few cars in the lot, someone would have coincidentally arrived just as she was walking out?
2. He was wearing sunglasses at night which means he was trying to conceal his identity. Cliché but true. This may also indicate he knew about the evidence camera and had planned to defeat it.
3. He wasn't carrying any of the things expected of someone intending to work out.
4. He began walking so they passed each other just as he got to the end of the car separating them. He perfectly timed his gait to be able to turn around closely behind her. Time between her spotting his car door open and him closing off her escape path was mere seconds.

Now let's examine her actions and what she might have done differently. Important note: *I'm not criticizing her. She wasn't at fault at all; she was simply not trained.* I wish I could have been there to escort her to her vehicle. I'm using this incident to point out how disadvantaged *any* untrained person is when confronted with an experienced predator.

1. She didn't project the image of a hard target—overtly watching him as he continued behind her. Even if her awareness and bold attitude hadn't deterred him, it may have afforded her time to flee or launch a preemptive counterattack.
2. Her body language revealed that she was clearly uncomfortable with

this individual. She didn't act on her gut feeling or her gut feeling didn't have enough time to kick in before he'd cut off her escape.

3. Not being trained to always have a plan (awareness, avoidance, fleeing…) means she needed to assess the situation and in a moment piece together those **Red Flag** clues to recognize the beginning of an attack. Then— while her cognitive skills were evaporating—she'd have had to make up a plan: fight or run. His careful planning *intentionally* robbed her of the time to analyze, decide, then act. Recall that your goal is to stay ahead of predators.

4. Very, very few if any untrained people would have escaped this attack— and not all trained people would have. A female black belt would have needed to fight ferociously against this large, brutal thug. His intended victim needed to have inviolable habits (rules) preset for herself to immediately flee threatening situations, or better yet to routinely request someone in the gym to escort her to her car after dark. These suggestions fit our Five Step Plan.

5. We all like to think "everyone is just like me", so we treat others, even strangers, with respect and a degree of *(dangerous) unearned trust.* We hesitate to keep a sharp eye on people nearby who could be threats. Predators plan on this, and often victims later confess in regret, "I knew something wasn't right about the guy, but I didn't want to offend anyone…" Had she turned around to observe any innocent passer-by, she would have only seen his back as he walked into the gym—and he wouldn't have known he was being observed. *The only person who'd notice that she'd turned around to monitor him would be someone who had turned around to watch her. There was no downside to overtly keeping him in sight.* In fact, such watchfulness would have announced that she was a hard target. **RUDE IS THE NEW SAFE.**

To survive and escape an attack with minimum injury, you need a plan as well as awareness of our common weaknesses and strengths.

Our Problems

"Everyone is just like me" mindset (puppy dog mode):

This is such a dangerous yet common mindset that I devote an entire chapter of this book to it.

Anxiety:

Is a sense of alarm about an *uncertain* threat that concerns the *future*. It arises from conflict—either internal ("I doubt my ability to handle this situation") or between you and the external ("Why is that man watching me?"). Anxiety can be paralyzing; at minimum it consumes some cognitive ability.

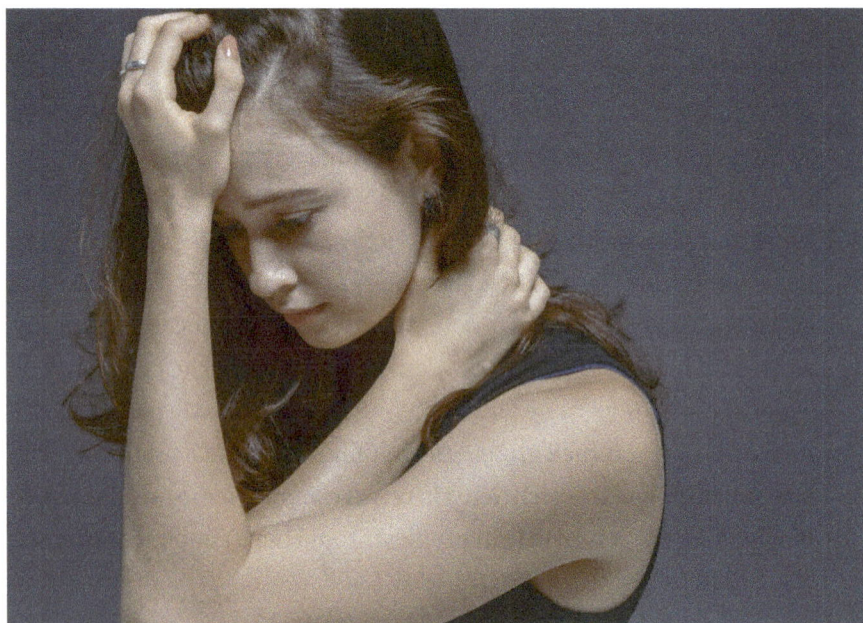

Photo: Ketut Subiyanto

Doubt/lack of confidence:

Doubt shoves confidence aside. Doubt can spring from a lack of training and practice.

Threat:

When referring to people, we mean a person we *suspect* has the *intent*, *opportunity*, and *ability and means* to do us harm. Situations in which attacks frequently occur are also threats. Fatigue or impairment by substances are threats for obvious reasons.

Bystander Effect:

Witnesses of an ongoing attack refuse to help the victim. The greater the number of passive witnesses, the more at ease they all feel about conforming with the crowd and not helping.[19]

Bandwagon Effect:

Believing something because others do.

Risk:

We feel at risk when we don't know what's going to happen. Risk is not just the *probability* of an event, it's also how serious the *consequences* could be.

Continuation Bias:

Wanting to continue on your original plan when it's no longer wise due to changed conditions. The young women in the opening story suffered from Continuation Bias. They kept walking toward their vehicle even after they noticed drunk males near it. (*"We've walked to our cars in dark parking lots many times and nothing bad has ever happened."*) This is such a dangerous mindset that pilots call it "get-home-itis" and train to avoid it.

Expectation Bias:

---

[19] "Bystander Effect: What Is Bystander Effect?" (accessed June 24, 2016); available from https://www.psychologytoday.com/basics/bystander-effect

You believe facts that align with your expectations but discard facts that do not. It arises from your belief that your "actions can produce a particular outcome."[20]

Confirmation Bias:

You interpret information in a way that confirms what you want to believe. Example: You've just met someone you want to like so you notice the nice things he does, but dismiss **Red Flags** in his behavior.[21]

Herding:

People in a group acting as one, without conscious direction or decisions, "often making decisions as a group that they would not make as an individual."[22]

Habits (Old): To streamline our lives, we outsource conscious thinking to habits. *If we're not disciplined we can allow old habits to override our gut feeling and awareness.* Think of habits as an autopilot that you need to keep an eye on because once in a while an autopilot as well as your habits can put you in a bad position.

Complacency (the killer):

Relaxing your attention below the level needed to ensure your safety because you've never had a problem in this situation before. Complacency can lead to many of the above problems. Symptoms: you fail to notice important things around you until they're a threat and you're OK with that or you abandon your safety plan when you know you shouldn't.

---

[20] Expectancy (accessed March 30, 2021); available from https://dictionary.apa.org/expectancy

[21] Confirmation bias (accessed March 30, 2021); available from https://dictionary.apa.org/confirmation-bias

[22] "Herd Behavior (Behavioral Economics)" (accessed March 30, 2020; available from https://www.tutor2u.net/economics/reference/behavioural-economics-herd-behaviour

You can see we humans come bundled with an odd set of conflicting software. We feel fear and anxiety that try to keep us safe, but we misuse the higher thinking part of our brains to overpower those healthy, gut instincts by selectively ignoring or dismissing clues that tell us we're getting into trouble. We need to be alert to this, and self-controlled.

Our Tools

Gut Feeling:

I list this one first because it doesn't require any preparation or training. You have it already. Your subconscious may notice something that your conscious (and perhaps distracted) mind misses—movement, unexpected sound, someone where they shouldn't be or doing something odd. It could be your subconscious mind metaphorically sticking an elbow into your conscious mind's ribs. Remember, after being attacked many victims report they'd had a gut feeling about the situation or person and regret not honoring it.

Mindset:

The defender's mindset is much like the pilot's mindset. This shared mindset includes a *measure of cynicism* and replaces hope with *planning* (including alternatives) and *practiced* skills. A defender's mindset requires *honest assessments* of one's abilities and the seriousness of any current Threats (**awareness**). The prudent pilot knows that any problems she doesn't find on the ground will find her in the air, so part of her job is to *identify (**awareness**) and leave problems behind (**avoidance**)*, on the ground or detour around threats in the air. She knows that a momentary lapse of attention can be dangerous, so she is *disciplined in her awareness.* She expects the best but is *constantly* planning for the current worst-case scenario given the existing dynamic situation. And she will *do whatever it takes* to bring her passengers, crew and aircraft home safely. What does this look like?

It might be simply *declining to participate*—what pilots call the "no-go" decision. Sometimes the captain or the sole pilot of a light aircraft (both are legally referred to as "pilot-in-command", or PIC) decides to wait until external circumstances change, such as weather that's expected to clear or a deferred-inoperative aircraft component is repaired or replaced (**avoidance**). The PIC might decide deviate more widely around growing enroute thunderstorms (**avoidance**, again) or to divert to an alternate airport if conditions deteriorate at the planned destination (**fleeing**). A destination is always a *planned* destination until landing there; *willingness to change your plans* is required (the equivalent of **complying** with demands of a Threat so as to prevent confrontation). The last step in our Five Step Plan, **(counter)attack**, is the equivalent of proficient flying skills to survive hazardous conditions. Pilots specifically use awareness and avoidance to prevent having to rely on sharp flying skills to **escape** threatening conditions.

Rude is the New Safe (i.e., "Everyone is *not* just like me"):

Honoring your gut feeling and sticking to your awareness and avoidance habits *will require you to break out of your comfort zone and be rude at times.* Your safety takes priority over other people's feelings. Overcoming a lifetime habit of assuming everyone you encounter lives by civilized rules requires *changing your mindset.* The scenarios you should practice that are described in the Pulling It All Together chapter will help you make the bold decisions you need to stay safe.

Habits (New):

Use the awareness and avoidance tips in this book to replace old habits. It is easier to replace a less helpful habit with a more helpful one than it is to simply quit with nothing in its place.

Plan:

Having a plan to work through during a stressful situation takes your mind away from the unknowable future (anxiety) and back to the present.

Fear:

Your emotional response to a *known* threat.[23] Fear—while no fun—keeps you in the present and activates your helpful (as well as not-so-helpful) survival responses.

Paying Attention and Training:

Identify potential *threats* and *resources*. In addition to your personal experience, paying attention includes your senses, reasoning, and gut feeling.

Risk Assessment:

Analysis of the *probability* and *consequences* of suspected threats acting.

Resources:

Helpers with you, nearby emergency responders, open businesses, crowds you can disappear into, legal weapons you have with you.

Security Layers:

Projecting the image of a hard target, listening to your gut, avoiding threats, bringing helpers, not becoming impaired, not being around people who are impaired, avoiding places or times that facilitate attacks, paying attention, and learning how to fight fulfill the goal of security layers. Most of these are simple steps. No single layer is sufficient, but together they provide more complete protection and make you a *hard target*. The usual visual aid is a pile of slices of Swiss cheese. Stack enough slices to leave no holes.

Hard Target:

A person who takes overt steps to improve his or her security. Visibly confident and aware, you want to project the image of a hard target in order to dissuade predators from approaching.

Stealth Fighting Stance:

---

[23] "What's the Difference Between Fear and Anxiety?" (accessed June 24, 2016); available from http://panicdisorder.about.com/od/understandingpanic/a/fearandanxiety.htm

Placing your hands between a Threat and your upper body and face (place the forearm of your arm closer to the Threat vertically with your chin in your hand and your other forearm across your midsection with your open hand over your floating rib) and turn slightly away to protect your vital organs along your center line. This is the so-called "Jack Benny" position, after the droll comedian who often stood in this pose. This is a non-obvious fighting position that allows you to protect and if necessary fight back quickly and unexpectedly, yet without appearing aggressive to a potential Threat.

Red Flag:

Something that may seem trivial but points to a bigger problem. Attempts by a male to get you to drink alcohol, separate you from the crowd (**Intoxicate & Isolate**), or persistently pry your personal information from you are Red Flags, as are men who disrespect women. A few seemingly small signals add up to one huge Red Flag. *A Red Flag tells you to reassess your situation and take steps to insure your safety.*

Plan:

This is a result of paying attention and your risk assessment (probability and consequences), with the goal of staying ahead of predators. A security plan might consider an entire international vacation, a night out, or the next few seconds. However, planning stops when violence begins.

Safety:

Safety not the absence of harm—especially in the short term. Safety is about controlling risk. A person who crosses a busy street blindfolded and somehow doesn't get run over is not safe, just lucky this time. Luck is not a plan.

Confidence:

Confidence shoves doubt aside. Having confidence also helps you project the image of a hard target, which makes you less likely to be accosted.

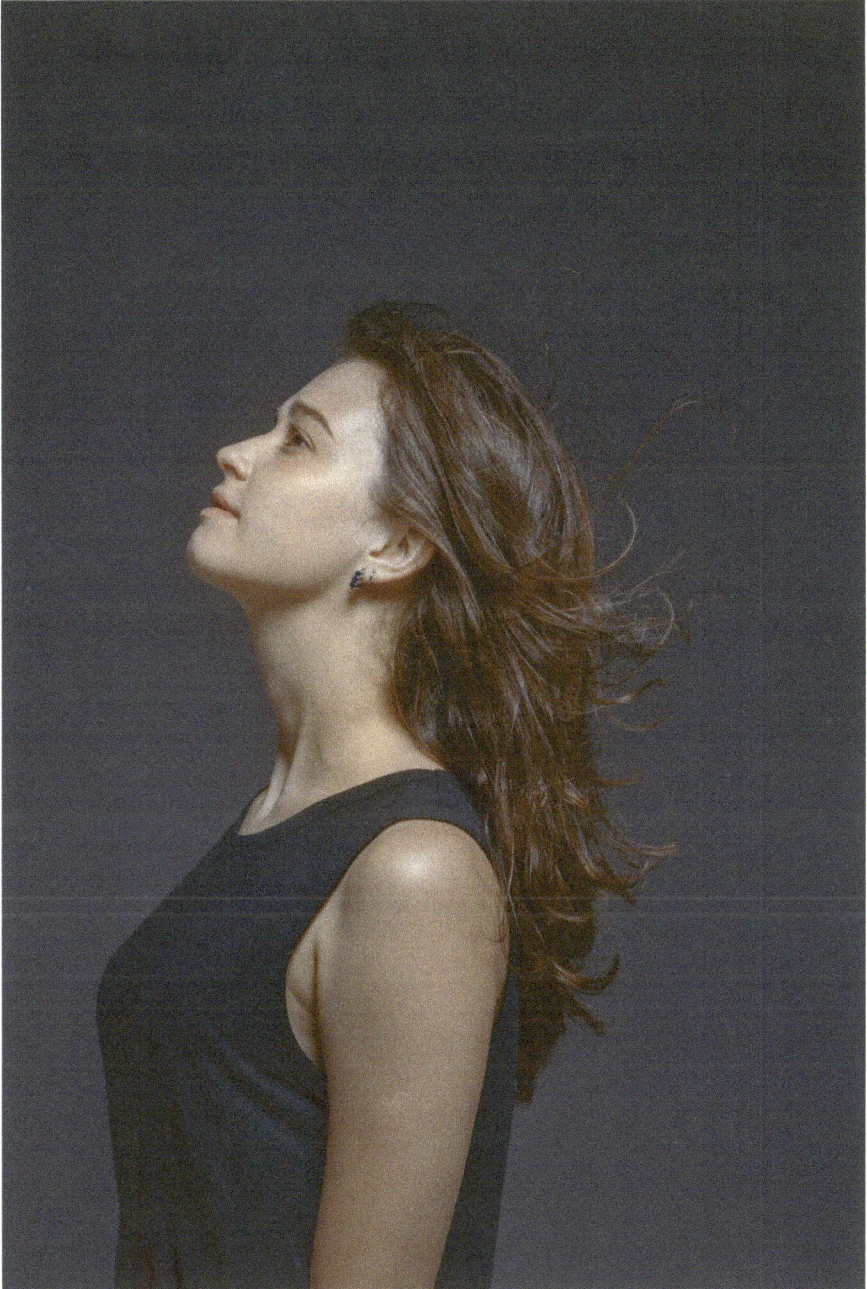

Photo: Ketut Subiyanto

* * *

Awareness: Kathy Long has been called the Queen of Mean. Five-time World Women's Kickboxing Champion, she is at this writing a mixed martial arts fighter in her fifties. Among other arts, she has trained in kickboxing and Brazilian Jiu Jitsu.

Let's see what she says about self-defense and paying attention to our environment: "It's essential to walk with confidence and keep your head up and your shoulders squared. Always scan your environment. When a predator sees that you're in touch with your surroundings, he's more likely to think 'She's a little too aware of what's going on. She doesn't look like the meek, mild, timid type. She doesn't look like the type who'll try to get into her car without paying attention.'"[24]

Check out this video[25] or do a search for "Kathy Long teaching self-defense" to see what a self-defense course taught by a world champion can look like.

---

[24] "6 Things You Need to Know About Self-defense — Advice From One of the Greatest Kickboxers in History!" (accessed May 5, 2016); available from http://www.blackbeltmag.com/daily/self-defense-training/6-things-you-need-to-know-about-self-defense-advice-from-one-of-the-greatest-kickboxers-in-history/

[25] "Kathy Long Teaching Urban Defense Tactics" (accessed November 10, 2023); available from https://www.youtube.com/watch?v=3alhMgvRaf0

6

RISK = PROBABILITY x CONSEQUENCES

"Now, you may think you don't work in a high-risk situation like a police officer or a bouncer, so you don't have to worry about being attacked, right? Wrong! Life is a high-risk situation. Prepare accordingly." —*"Sensei Ando" Mierzwa*[26]

---

[26] Ando Mierzwa "Defense Against A Sucker Punch" (accessed April 19, 2020); available from https://www.youtube.com/watch?v=qJLdXitWlaI

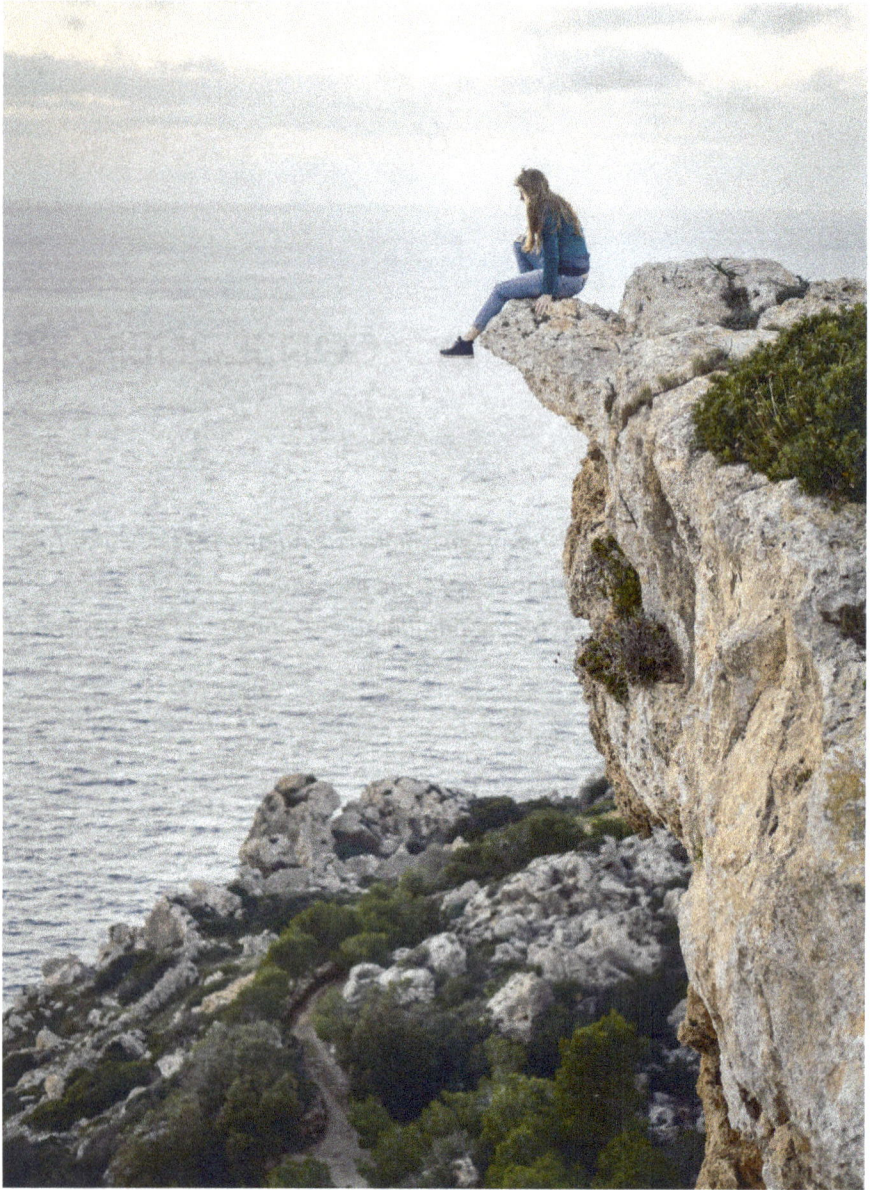

Photo: Lukas Hartmann

How fast can a friendly get-together turn into a potential sexual assault?

While at a gathering of acquaintances in a home, a very intoxicated woman unwittingly made clear to everyone present that she was sexually available for the evening. No takers. She eventually passed out, after which a short but serious conversation ensued about whether someone might take her up on her availability—while she was unconscious. Just..like...that.

- If you could have asked that woman she would have told you that all the people there were "friends"—*a recklessly overused word.* She never found out that someone had brought up that she could be sexually assaulted while unconscious. Clearly that would never have been thought, much less spoken, by real friends.
- Recall that safety is about managing risk. This young woman made herself vulnerable in **the number-one situation for sexual assaults on college-age women: a residence with drinking males she already knew**. By luck, she woke up the following morning unharmed except for a hangover—and ignorance of the previous night's danger. Luck is not a plan.
- Last point: Her behavior told everyone there (and those they might later speak to) that all someone has to do to get her into bed is pour enough alcohol down her throat. One evening of bad judgment can echo for a long time.

Risk: Probability

According to a 2014 Department of Justice, Bureau of Justice Statistics (BJS) Special Report, "Rape and Sexual Assault Victimization Among College-Age Females, 1995–2013," college-age women who were victims of sexual assault and rape knew the offender in eight of ten crimes.[27],[28] Half the students were attacked by "friends or acquaintances." In other words: **most college-age women who are attacked know their attackers but don't realize what these men are capable of.**

About half of the female students in the study were attacked while engaged in leisurely activities away from their homes, while roughly half of non-student women were accosted while at home. About two-thirds of all attacks occurred between the hours of six o'clock PM and six o'clock AM.[29]

The most common venues for rape and sexual assaults against women ages 18-24: in or near the residence of the victim or of a relative/friend/acquaintance of victim (67%), commercial places including parking lots and garages (15-16%), and open public areas including public transportation, parks and playgrounds (13-16%). The varying occurrence ranges are due to different statistics for students than for non students in this age group.[30],[31] Even when you're in a home where you're comfortable you should not lower your attention or fail to follow the steps you're learning.

"Two people are charged in connection with the rape of a 15-year-old girl at a

---

[27] Sofi Sinozich, and Lynn Langton, Ph.D., "Rape and Sexual Assault Victimization Among College-Age Females, 1995–2013" Bureau of Justice Statistics, Office of Justice Programs, US Department of Justice, December, 2014:7

[28] If we assume that most women would not knowingly associate with men whom they suspect might attack them, then we see that 80% of sexual assault victims misjudged the character of their male associates, or didn't take seriously clues that the males around them were capable of violence. In other words, *some women—you?—are now associating with men who will someday attack them*. The lesson here is not to try to get better at judging people, but to not put yourself in situations that would give someone the opportunity to assault you.

[29] Sofi Sinozich, and Lynn Langton, Ph.D.,:6

[30] *Ibid.*

[31] Greenfield, Lawrence A. 1997. Sex Offenses and Offenders: An Analysis of Data on Rape and Sexual Assault, Washington, DC: Bureau of Justice Statistics, Office of Justice Programs, US Department of Justice.

home..."[32]

The most common places for violent crimes against males and females of all ages are: on or near your property (33.7%), on a street other than near your residence or residence of relative/friend/acquaintance (14%), school (through high school) property (13%), commercial locations such as restaurants, bars and nightclubs or other commercial buildings (12%), at or near home of relative, friend or neighbor (9%), and parking lots and garages (7%). The most common venues for property crimes: at or near home of victim (60%), parking lots and garages (11%), school property (7%) and commercial locations (5%).[33] Note that 14% of violent crimes but only 2.5% of property crimes occur on a street other than near your residence or residence of relative/friend/acquaintance.

Unfortunately, statistics for sexual crimes vary widely, because of differing definitions used or survey methodologies. As an example, one study claimed that one in five college women are victims of sexual assault or rape during their college years. Bureau of Justice Statistics (considered authoritative) indicates that one in 52.6 college women will be victims of sexual assault or rape during their college years.[34] While not the shocking one-in-five, that is still an alarming number. To put that into perspective: in any group of 5,260 women tracked during their four college years, 100 of them will be raped or sexually assaulted. Statistically, then, during an academic year on a coed campus of around 10,000 students, 100 women will be sexually assaulted or raped. That makes **one woman attacked every three days** during Fall and Spring semesters. It can't happen to you?

---

[32] "Two charged in rape of teen in Salisbury" (accessed on January 9, 2016); available from http://www.delmarvanow.com/story/news/local/maryland/2015/11/02/two-charged-rape-teen-salisbury/75050264/

[33] "Location," Bureau of Justice Statistics, Office of Justice Programs, US Department of Justice, 2008.:1 Available from https://www.bjs.gov/index.cfm?ty=tp&tid=44. Note this data is from 2008.

[34] "Are 1 In 5 Women Raped In College?" (accessed April 29, 2016); available from https://www.prageru.com/courses/political-science/are-1-5-women-raped-college

Keep that number in mind as you look over the following statistics that were collected by the National Sexual Violence Resource Center's *Sexual Assault Statistics* paper that quotes from numerous studies.

- *Approximately eight of ten rapes are committed by someone the victim knows.*[35,36] Think about the get-together I just described.
- *More than 6 of 10 rape victims are between the ages of 12 and 24.*[37] A possible contributing factor is that young, single people tend to move around and exercise outdoors alone, stay out late and those of drinking age frequent places where alcohol is being used. That lifestyle puts them in harm's way, calling for honed survival skills.

According to HomeFacts.com, as of April 2021, 347 registered sex offenders live in my county of approximately 260,000 residents. Since registered sex offenders are virtually all male, this comes out to three of every thousand males in this county.

About the University of Maryland: "*From July 2014 through June 30 [2015], the [Office of Student Conduct] fully investigated 13 of 48 complaints, including seven cases of Sexual Assault I (nonconsensual penetration), three stalking and sexual harassment cases, two sexual harassment cases and one relationship violence*

---

[35] Greenfield, Lawrence A.

[36] Tjaden, Patricia, Thoennes, Nancy. November 1998. "Full Report of the Prevalence, Incidence, and Consequences of Violence Against Women: Findings from the National Violence Against Women Survey," Washington (DC): National Institute of Justice, Office of Justice Programs, US Department of Justice. Report NCJ 183781

[37] *Ibid.*

case."[38]

Maybe those numbers don't sound high but keep in mind that up to 80% of sexual assaults on college women go unreported.[39]

Statistics lose meaning when you are the victim.

Instant Predator: Just Add Alcohol

According to the Sinozich and Langton study,[40] nearly half of sexual assault victims believed their attackers had been drinking. Alcohol use—by either the victim or attacker—is a factor in many rape cases.

We Resident Assistants in my coed dorm during my senior year of college were kept informed about incidents across campus. Friday and Saturday nights make up only a few of the 168 hours in a week, but at nearly all of the problems that occurred on campus happened during those short times when alcohol flows freely.

Not becoming impaired, not being around people who are getting impaired, and avoiding males who are impulsive, violent or disrespect women even in little things, are free and simple security layers for you.

Lifeboat Crowders

Women and children ~~first~~ *get out of my way.*

According to a Swedish study of maritime catastrophes, "Out of the 15,142

---

[38] "University of Maryland Expels Record Number Of Students For Sexual Assault" (accessed January 1, 2016); available from http://www.diamondbackonline.com/news/university-of -maryland-expels-record-number-of-students-for-sexual/article_944bab50-8747-11e 5-866f-ab4d62e2c4dd.html. Of the 35 cases the office did not fully investigate, 15 were voluntarily resolved, in 10 cases the filer declined to continue the complaint, 6 were pending investigation, 3 cases lacked evidence and 1 case was not sexual misconduct. Three expulsions, a record number, resulted.

[39] Sofi Sinozich, and Lynn Langton, Ph.D. :1

[40] Sofi Sinozich, and Lynn Langton, Ph.D.:18

people onboard the 18 ships sailing under eight different national flags when they went down, only 17.8 percent of the women survived compared to 34.5 percent of the men, the two researchers explain in their 82-page study titled: 'Every man for himself—Gender, Norms and Survival in Maritime Disasters.'"

The researchers cite the passenger ferry *Estonia*, which sank on a run from Tallinn, Estonia to Stockholm, Sweden in the cold Baltic Sea in 1994. Only about 5% of the women survived compared to 22% of the men.

The only "women and children first" exceptions the researchers found were the sinking of the British ships *Birkenhead* (1852) and *Titanic* (1912).[41] None in the past 100 years!

On January 13, 2012, the *Costa Concordia* cruise ship sank off the coast of Tuscany, Italy, killing 32 people. According to the English *Daily Mail*, "Fights broke out to get into the lifeboats, men refused to prioritize women, expectant mothers and children as they pushed themselves forward to escape" and, "survivors tell of panic as men ignore order that women and children should go first and passengers fight to get on boats."[42]

Men will *not* necessarily help you just because you're a woman.

Bystander Effect

Without helpers, you are on your own.[43] Recall from the Problems discussion in the Challenges & Tools chapter that the greater the number of witnesses to an attack, the likelihood of them helping you dwindles.

You need to be *prepared* and *able* to fend for yourself.

---

[41] "Chivalry at sea a 'myth', Swedish study shows" (accessed February 3, 2016); available from http://phys.org/news/2012-04-chivalry-sea-myth-swedish.html

[42] "Swim ahead, darling, I'll survive: 'My husband gave me his lifejacket as we jumped off sinking cruise ship... I never saw him again,' says French survivor (accessed February 3, 2016); available from http://www.dailymail.co.uk/news/article-2086826/Costa-Concordia-cruise-ship-accident-French-survivor-tells-husband-gave-lifejacket.html

[43] "Bystander Effect" (accessed January 20, 2016); available from https://www.psychologytoday.com/basics/bystander-effect

Risk: Consequences

"The price of preparation and surety is inconsequential when compared to the cost of failure and tragedy." —Edward Wilks

According to HelpGuide.org, "Traumatic experiences often involve a threat to life or safety...The more frightened and helpless you feel, the more likely you are to be traumatized."[44] As you recall from the Challenges & Tools chapter, the degree to which a physical attack triggers your sympathetic nervous system—which affects your ability to fight back—can be lessened by training to avoid or meet violence. *Awareness and avoidance training makes you less likely to be targeted for an attack and fighting training can make you more likely to be able to escape.*

In addition to possible long-term physical injuries, a sexual attack can result in immediate ("shock, disbelief, denial, fear, confusion, anxiety, and withdrawal") and long-term psychological trouble, such as PTSD that can linger for months or longer. Other long-term effects include "anxiety, substance abuse, sleep disturbances, depression, alienation, and sexual dysfunction." As if those problems aren't enough, a risk factor for sexual attack is a history of being sexual attacked; survivors have an increased likelihood of being attacked again. They are also more likely to take part in risky sexual behavior and are more prone to try or commit suicide than non-victims.[45]

---

[44] "Emotional and Psychological Trauma" (accessed February 8, 2016); available from http://ww w.helpguide.org/articles/ptsd-trauma/emotional-and-psychological-trauma.htm

[45] Riviello, Ralph J., MD, FACEP. "Evaluating and Treating Sexual Assault in the Emergency Department." Emergency Medicine Reports, August 21, 2005. Relias Media. Available from https://www.reliasmedia.com/articles/83668-evaluating-and-treating-sexual-assault-in -the-emergency-department

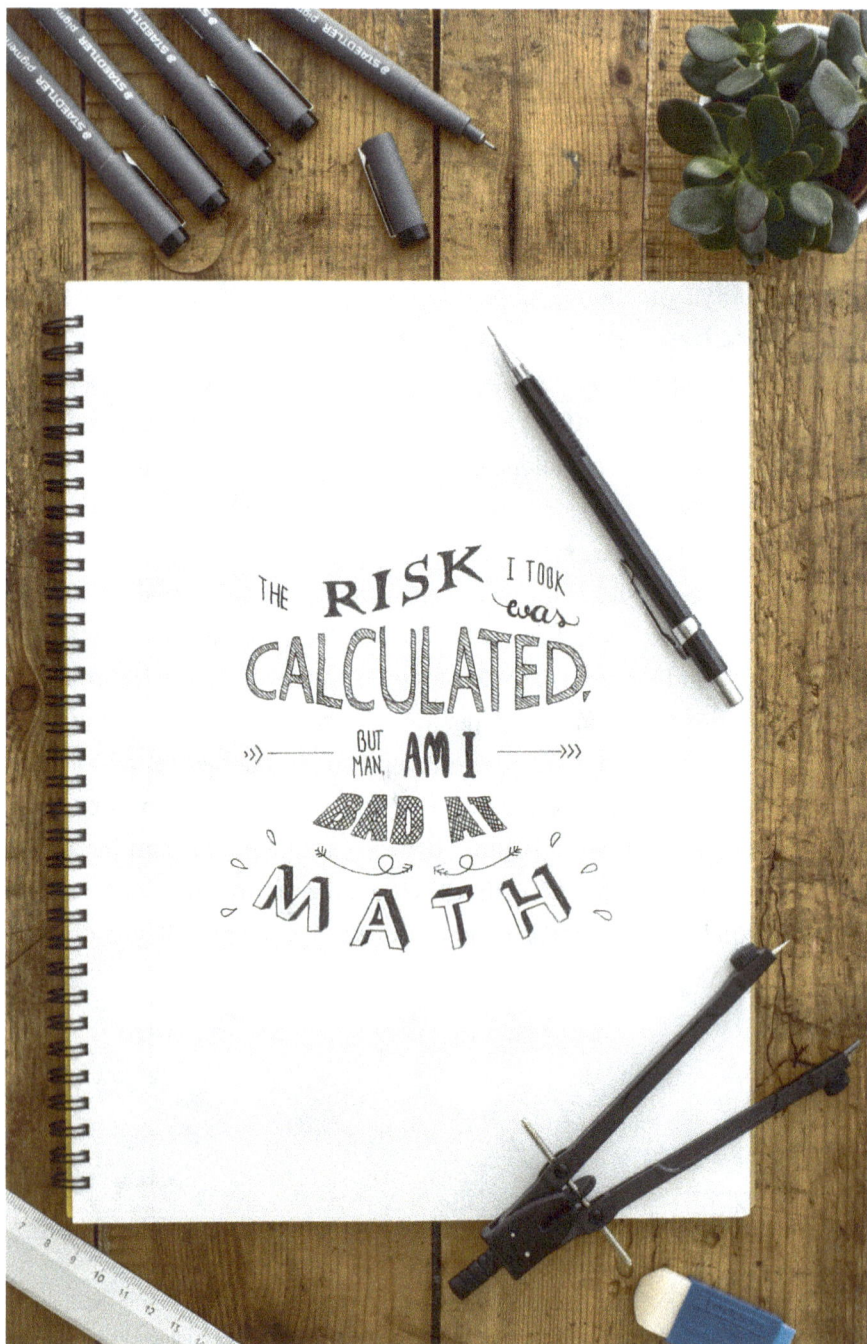

Photo: lum3n

* * *

Some people think Benny "The Jet" Urquidez is the best full contact fighter of all time. No wonder, he has over sixty professional victories, has won titles in several weight classes and is undefeated in defending his world championship titles over decades. Today, he still trains and teaches. He very clearly understands the mental as well as physical aspects of fighting.

In this video[46], he tells us his Five Rules of Training.

---

[46] Benny The Jet's Five Rules of Training: https://www.youtube.com/watch?v=QIq0ElVe8LY

7

BE READY TO AVOID VIOLENCE

"The will to succeed is important, but what's more important is the will to prepare." —*Coach Bobby Knight*

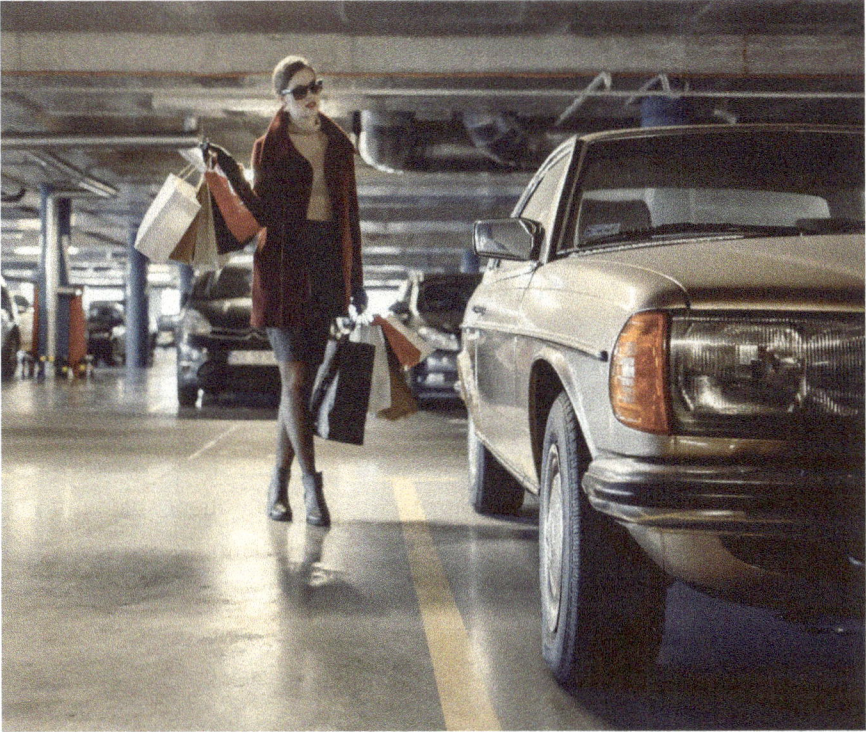

If approached by a robber, this woman should be ready to toss her valuables to divert the predator's attention away from her and possibly allow her a safe escape.
Photo: freestockorg

H ope Is Not A Plan.

We've examined the probabilities and consequences of assaults. Who are committing these crimes?

A man from Glen Burnie, Maryland "was charged with first-, second-, third- and fourth-degree sex offenses, along with first- and second-degree assault..."[47]

Risk factors increasing the likelihood that a man will commit sexual assault can be organized into four categories: individual, relationship, community and societal. These factors include: alcohol or drug use, impulsiveness, anger toward women, poor family environment, sexually aggressive associates, and tolerance of sexual assault in their community or society.[48]

The Attacker's Toolbox

- Unreported or unprosecuted "rapists are extremely adept at identifying 'likely' victims, and testing prospective victims' boundaries
- "Plan and premeditate their attacks, using sophisticated strategies to groom their victims for attack, and to isolate them physically
- "Use 'instrumental', non-gratuitous violence; they exhibit strong impulse control and use only as much violence as is needed to terrify and coerce their victims into submission
- "Use psychological weapons: power, control, manipulation, and threats – backed up by physical force, and almost never resort to weapons such as knives or guns
- "Use alcohol deliberately to render victims more vulnerable to attack, or completely unconscious.
- "In addition, the majority of undetected rapists are serial rapists who also commit other forms of serious interpersonal violence."[49]

In fact, in the study referred to above, the author said that these stealth rapists

---

[47] "Police charge man with third sexual assault in Glen Burnie" (accessed January 1, 2016); available from http://www.capitalgazette.com/news/for_the_record/ph-ac-cn-sexual-assault-charges-1114-20151113-story.html

[48] Riviello, Ralph J., MD, FACEP

[49] "Rape Fact Sheet," David Lysak, Ph.D., 2002, University of Massachusetts Boston. Found at http://www.binghamton.edu/counseling/documents/RAPE_FACT_SHEET1.pdf

frequently use alcohol as a weapon in their crimes. He also characterized these males as very sexually active and being angry at women. They picture women as conquests and themselves as super-masculine.[50]

"Months after a college student was raped by a friend at a party she hosted, *it continues to affect her life,* a prosecutor said Friday [emphasis added]."[51]

"An 18-year-old [male] Virginia Tech student has been charged with murder after the remains of a 13-year-old Blacksburg girl missing since Wednesday were found in Surry County, North Carolina, Blacksburg Police Chief Anthony Wilson announced at a news conference Saturday night...[the 13 year old girl] was active on social media, participating in several 'teen dating' Facebook groups."[52] And later, *"A second Virginia Tech student was arrested Sunday in connection with the death of a 13-year-old girl who disappeared last week. Police said [a woman] helped dispose of the girl's body, which was found by police Saturday in North Carolina. Virginia Tech confirmed she was a sophomore at the school."[53]* Not all predators are male.

You cannot "meet" or "know" people online—or even over the phone. Most information transfer is nonverbal, and that is missing from texts, emails, and most other forms of electronic conversation. When you look at a person's social media pages, the only things you see about him are what he chooses to display—and those factors may not be true. Think about the cheating, arrests,

---

[50] The Undetected Rapist," David Lysak, Ph.D., 2002, University of Massachusetts Boston. Found at http://www.binghamton.edu/counseling/documents/RAPE_FACT_SHEET1.pdf"

[51] "Man gets 20 years in rape of college student at party" (accessed January 9, 2016); available from http://www.delmarvanow.com/story/news/local/maryland/2015/09/18/salisbury-party-rape/72396770/

[52] "Missing Blacksburg girl found dead, police announce" (accessed February 3, 2016); available from http://www.roanoke.com/news/local/blacksburg/missing-blacksburg-girl-found-dead-police-announce/article_aaffb7cb-328a-5bd0-9555-14c6a78f1f19.html

[53] "Second Virginia Tech student arrested in death of missing 13-year-old girl" (accessed February 3, 2016); available from http://www.foxnews.com/us/2016/01/31/virginia-tech-student-arrested-in-death-missing-teen.html

STAYING SAFE FOR TODAY'S WOMAN

child and substance abuse and other icky things reported about celebrities in the press. Now imagine how different your image of those same people would be if your only sources were their sanitized social media pages. It is possible that you know more about a distant celebrity than a nearby neighbor.

What About The Mentally Ill?

My purpose in this section is to expose you to certain *observable behaviors* so that you might earlier recognize them as *possible* **Red Flags**—whether warning you of violent outbursts or people who would manipulate you. I am NOT trying to teach you how to diagnose disorders—something I am not qualified to do. A selfish person can display some of these behaviors: no matter, avoid those people, too. You may find that people who display these behaviors trigger your gut feeling—and you know what to do when that happens.

This is not an exhaustive examination of violence committed by mentally ill persons. In 2015 a meta study of studies was conducted on violence perpetrated by people with mental disorders. The study showed that people with serious mental illness are victimized more often than they commit violence, and that people with serious mental illness *who are receiving effective treatment* are no more dangerous than people not mentally ill. However, many of the studies examined found that people with serious mental illness who were not being treated effectively, or were not complying with medication instructions, or were abusing alcohol or drugs did commit violent crimes at much higher rates than people not mentally ill.[54] This conclusion was also reached in a 2010 Swedish study of violent crimes committed by people with bipolar disorder: violence above the rate committed by non-mentally ill

---

[54] Swanson, J.W., McGinty, E.E., Fazel, S., Mays, V.M. (2015). Mental illness and reduction of gun violence and suicide: Bringing epidemiologic research to policy. Annals of Epidemiology, 25, 366–376.

persons was attributed to concurrent substance abuse.[55]

Similarly, "Schizophrenic patients have less insight, experience greater thought disorder, and have poorer control of their aggressive impulses. Comorbidity with alcohol or other substances of abuse is frequent and complicates the agitation and the impulsivity. Among patients with schizophrenia, MDD [Major Depressive Disorder], and bipolar disorder, the risk for homicide was found to be increased with comorbid alcohol abuse or dependence." Multiple factors affect aggressive behavior, and the chance of violent outbursts is worse within a few months of being discharged from residential care.[56]

People with depression and anxiety disorders can exhibit excessive aggression and violence, which "likely develop as a consequence of generally disturbed emotional regulation, such as abnormally high or low levels of anxiety." Also, persons with depression commit impulsive-reactive aggression, while patients with antisocial personality disorder (see below) display controlled-proactive aggression.[57]

You may not discern whether someone suffers from depression, anxiety, or personality disorders, but remember, you're not trying to diagnose or make excuses for these behaviors. Your job is to avoid threats by recognizing and moving away from them.

Sociopathy and psychopathy are not official psychological diagnoses. Their symptoms are grouped under Antisocial Personality Disorder, APD. Nevertheless sociopaths and psychopaths are commonly discussed. They, along with narcissists (people with Narcissistic Personalty Disorder, NPD), fall under Cluster B of the *Diagnostic and Statistical Manual of Mental Disorders,* or *DSM-5.*

---

[55] "Bipolar disorder does not increase risk of violent crime, Swedish study suggests" (accessed April 10, 2021); available from https://www.sciencedaily.com/releases/2010/09/1009071036 13.htm

[56] "Aggression and Impulsivity in Schizophrenia" (accessed April 10, 2021); available from https://www.psychiatrictimes.com/view/aggression-and-impulsivity-schizophrenia

[57] Inga D. Neumann, Alexa H. Veenema, and Daniela I. Beiderbecke, "Aggression and Anxiety: Social Context and Neurobiological Links" *Frontiers in Behavioral Neuroscience*, US National Library of Medicine, National Institutes of Health, March, 2010.:4, 12

People with APD show a lack of empathy and regard for others and don't care about right and wrong. They are unable to have emotionally intimate relationships. They may engage in aggressive or violent behavior—although most people with APD are not violent. However, they will go to extremes to get people to do their bidding, including lying, manipulating, and even frightening them.

While sociopaths and psychopaths share traits and the terms are sometimes used interchangeably, some professionals distinguish between the two; often the main determinant used is severity. For instance, while psychopaths have no conscience, sociopaths have a weak conscience. Sociopaths may form weak relationships while psychopaths cannot. Sociopaths may recognize what they're doing but they rationalize it and don't care; psychopaths are unaware they've hurt others. Also, sociopaths can be hot-headed, impulsive and, when their behavior is challenged, fly off the handle with rage, while psychopaths tend to be ice-cold. Psychopaths can carry on what appears to be a normal life to cover for a life of crime. Speaking of crime, "the more a psychopath feels socially isolated, sad, and alone, the higher his or her risk for violence and impulsive and/or reckless behavior."[58]

Psychopaths may engage in promiscuous sexual behavior.[59] "They don't fear the consequences of their actions."[60] Psychopathy is more common among men than women.[61]

Roughly 5% of people have NPD, and they take care of their needs but are disinterested in anyone else's. He or she also can: lie often, use people

---

[58] "How Sociopaths are Different from Psychopaths" (accessed April 9, 2021); available from https://www.verywellmind.com/what-is-a-sociopath-380184

[59] "What is a Psychopath?" (accessed April 9, 2012); available from https://www.verywellmind.com/what-is-a-psychopath-5025217#citation-3

[60] "Sociopath v. Psychopath: What's the Difference?" (accessed April 9, 2021); available from https://www.webmd.com/mental-health/features/sociopath-psychopath-difference

[61] "Psychopath" (accessed April 9, 2021); available from https://www.healthline.com/health/psychopath

to achieve goals,[62] lack empathy for others, feel superior, believe he is special and entitled, be arrogant, or have an exaggerated view of her or his importance.[63]

Narcissism may come in two flavors, the more obvious being: "Grandiose, overt narcissism is characterized by boldness, arrogance, and grandiose personality traits. People with this type of NPD are more likely to lack empathy, behave aggressively, exploit others, have only weak emotional relationships, and engage in exhibitionist behaviors." The other type: "Vulnerable, covert narcissism is characterized by hypersensitivity and defensiveness."[64]

If you cannot escape a narcissist or sociopath, you need to establish and ruthlessly enforce granite-hard boundaries.

Sociopaths' lies, manipulations and abuses are intentional and they understand they are hurting people. They do not care.

You can see the threads running though some of the disorders discussed are a lack of empathy, feeling of entitlement, no regard for others, possible aggressive, impulsive, angry or violent (proactive or reactive) behavior, mood swings, poorly modulated emotions, a willingness to manipulate or otherwise take advantage of others, and frequent lying. Be alert for such behaviors that can be **Red Flags**, not to mention such people are stressful to be around and who needs that?

Real-Life Threats

The following discussion is by no means the complete list of threatening situations and tactics. Predators will continue to find new ways to attack. Our

---

[62] "Narcissistic Personality Disorder" (accessed April 9, 2021); available from https://my.clevel andclinic.org/health/diseases/9742-narcissistic-personality-disorder

[63] "Narcissistic Personality Disorder and Borderline Personality" (accessed April 9, 2021); available from https://www.verywellmind.com/narcissistic-personality-disorder-425426

[64] "What is Narcissistic Personality Disorder (NPD)?" (accessed April 9, 2021); available from https://www.verywellmind.com/what-is-narcissistic-personality-disorder-2795446#cit ation-7

Athena Women training course crafts common types of assaults into training scenarios to better prepare you to recognize and respond to these scenarios.

A particularly dangerous type of attack is when a victim is arriving home and an assailant follows and forces her inside by attacking her from behind while she is unlocking her door. A similar attack is when the home invader breaks into a female's residence and awaits her return. He may also ring the doorbell and wait for the victim to open the door for him. When inside with the victim, the locks on her doors now protect the attacker from anyone who might intervene. Ironically, attacks perpetrated by assailants who wait for victims on remote hiking or exercise paths are similar to home invasion attacks in that, contrary to most assaults, time is the predator's friend and the defender's enemy. *These predators are patient, expend considerable time and energy planning and waiting for their victims and are often **especially savage and violent**.*

As previously mentioned, the most common sexual assault is the known assailant attacking his victim during gatherings, especially where alcohol is consumed. The predator becomes impaired, or encourages the intended victim to consume in excess, or drops a drug into her drink. He gets a woman alone and sexually attacks her (**Intoxicate & Isolate**).

The drugged drink works even against college-educated, high functioning, professional women in public places; no one is immune, *not even you*. The attacker is more skilled at his game than you at parrying him. If his offense doesn't work, he just walks away. If your defense doesn't work, you wake up naked the next morning with no memory of how you got in that position. Pay attention, keep your mental and physical guard up, watch the mixing and pouring of beverages and ensure they're continuously covered. Do not allow anyone to hand you an open beverage, because if your BFF bought the drinks and didn't ruthlessly guard them, they could be spiked. If your drink is uncovered even for a moment, it's no longer yours. Predators know how to prey.

You should immediately get away from any male who seems determined to get you alone or pour alcohol down your throat. Get away *now*, before the alcohol lowers your alertness. Some bars used to have a "two drink minimum"; you should have a carved-in-stone *maximum* number and type of drinks when in public. How many? No more than what keeps you legal and safe to drive.

According to police, most attacks by males against females are sexual in nature, and those committed by strangers often occur from behind so as to take her by surprise.

Use caution when exercising outdoors—anywhere. When you are alone in the dark, you make an attack easy. Likewise, you are putting yourself at greater risk by using earphones, marking you as an unaware victim and rendering you unable to hear someone running up behind you.

Attackers bent on sexual assault grab their victims and take them to the ground or drag them to a second location (second crime scene) for the assault. Unspeakable things occur at second crime scenes. You *must not* allow yourself to be forced into a vehicle or forcibly moved to an out-of-sight location during an attack. *Consider being forcibly relocated a life-threatening emergency.* A restraining move (grab) by an assailant can be the first step to relocating you. Do not delay or mitigate your escape techniques. This is why you should learn escapes, including wrist releases, that work against an attacker who is trying to drag you away rather than techniques that look cool but only work if your assailant is stationary.

Avoid anyone concealing his face by wearing sunglasses after dark or with a hoody, low hat, or scarf; these are signs of someone who doesn't want to be identified.

Victims are commonly confronted by thugs who distract with conversation, then attack with strikes to the face (or strikes by an accomplice who approaches from behind) as part of a violent robbery.

Another common distraction scheme is asking the intended victim for the time, which distracts him or her. Since most of us now keep time with our cell phones, this also reveals to the predator whether the victim's device is worth stealing. This is such a common beginning to muggings that in some high-crime areas, victims begin handing over their valuables as soon as they're asked what time it is!

Attacks have also occurred on sidewalks and along roads during daylight hours. One particular tactic is a predator who engages a victim who is walking in the opposite direction in a moment of small talk. He then turns away and appears to be continuing his walk. As soon as the woman turns her back to him, he spins around and attacks. By talking with her, he succeeds in slowing or stopping her. His friendly greeting relaxes her attention level and she turns her back when she should be keeping an eye on him. Predators count on our politeness to deter us from overtly observing them with suspicion. **Rude is the new safe.**

Don't be the last to leave parties, bars, restaurants or shopping areas; travel in groups. Park close to store entrances and under lights. Drive each other to your cars.

Some physical attacks predators use:

From behind: snatching your belongings, choke, hair pull, clothing grab, wrist grab, bear hug. These maneuvers can be used to restrain or take the victim to the ground. And, as mentioned earlier, tackle from behind.

From in front or beside you: sucker punch plus the above attacks.

In broad daylight, a mugger can attack a woman from behind as she loads possessions into her car. His accomplice waits in a nearby car and swoops in to pick up the mugger as soon as the robbery is complete.

Reminder: Common high-risk situations include

- Not paying *attention* or
- Being *alone* or
- *Alcohol* consumption (by the victim and/or attacker)

The three As; the last two can occur as the Isolate & Intoxicate attack (three As and two Is).

Attacks often involve predators exploiting the admirable human traits of politeness and helping others. They try to use the best of ourselves against us.

One thing that might be too obvious to notice:

For a crook to steal expensive things, he must go where expensive items are. That means nicer shopping areas, business districts, and neighborhoods. Also, criminals adapt. For example, when cars became more difficult to steal due to electronically coded keys, car thieves changed their tactic to carjacking.

An important note:

Police want you to report attacks. They know and respect that sexual attacks are especially emotionally and psychologically devastating. If you're a minor and you're assaulted in any way, immediately tell your parents. Adults: don't delay reporting to the police. If you're in a place with its own security force, report the incident to them and don't let anyone talk you out of reporting any attack, attempted attack or suspicious activity to sworn law enforcement officers. The more information the police have, the better they pinpoint patrols to deter further attacks.

All-Important Mindset for Fighting Back

Yes, you can train your body to work differently, but neither teacher nor student can succeed in their joint goal without your mind on board. A key part of good physical training is to encourage your self-protection mindset.

Some of our students demonstrated to us the importance of mindset. These students (teenagers and adults with no prior fighting training), became astonishingly proficient fighters during their few sessions with us. This was because they arrived at the studio for their first lesson with strong self-protection mindsets. They had already set their intentions and understood at a visceral level that they were worth aggressively fighting for. Their hearts and heads were "all-in" from day one, so they were able to absorb the most from each training minute. By telling themselves that they were ready to fight, they got their subconscious minds on their side. Do not underestimate the importance of that (more on your subconscious ahead).

The goal of learning is to change behavior and responses and your head has to be in the game to let that happen.

A self-defense mindset means you are convinced that:

- Legally justifiable use of force against another person in your defense is moral and just.
- You are worth fighting back for, and you *will* if justified.

Take Initiative

"There are old pilots and there are bold pilots, but there are no old *and* bold pilots." This is an old aviation saw about cautious decision-making. Avoidance calls for a cynical mindset. The stereotype of a seasoned airline captain is a stubborn, even brusque character who says "no" a lot because he's seen it all and he doesn't let anyone talk him into cutting corners. Practice saying the lifesaving words **"No"**, **"Stop"**, and **"Wait"**—and enforcing them. Practice being rude. Practice not trying to solve everyone's problems. *Practice*.

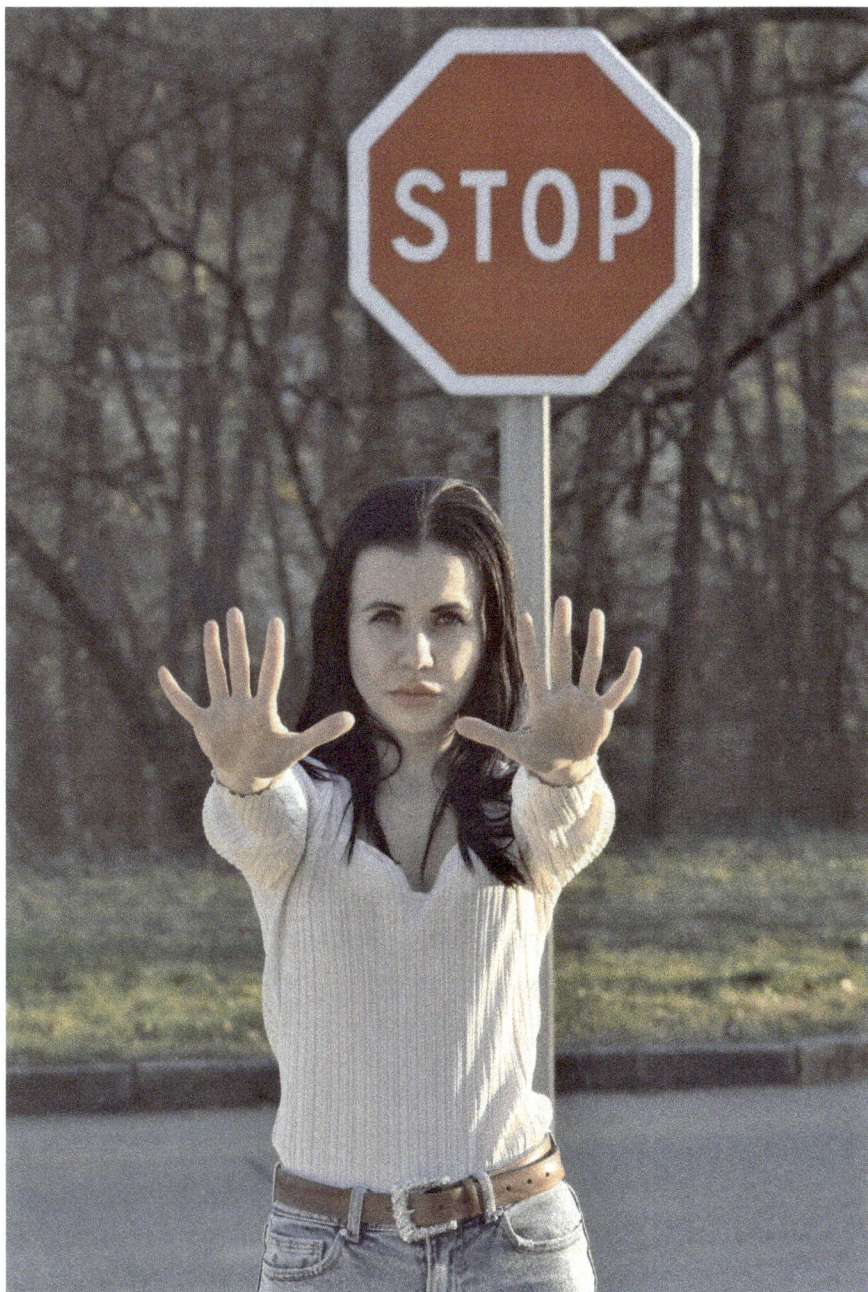

Photo: Daniele-la-Rosa-Messina

In an organization working toward a common goal, any *leadership* vacuum will be filled—and not always by the best candidate. Be deliberate about whom you follow. It's also true that when people are working at cross-purposes, any *power* vacuum will be filled— e.g. someone will seize power then exercise initiative to put his personal plan into action. Learning how to be proactive (**no, stop, wait**) in conflict situations can return power to you and keep you ahead of or away from a predator.

Remember the advice General James Mattis gave to his troops in Iraq: "Be polite, be professional, but have a plan to kill everybody you meet."[65]

This is an example of awareness and readiness in a war zone, but the attitude of awareness and planning is correct for all of us. You should have a plan to fight back and escape when you're in public. Make an *"if, then"* game out of it (*If* this man walks toward me, *then* I will...).

Acting from power doesn't mean that the predator suddenly fears you just because you wish that was the case.

Acting from power means you take initiative according to your Five Step Plan. This means taking verbal or some type of physical action (such as fleeing or preparing to fight) as opposed to waiting to react during a situation that is becoming more dangerous by the second. You are not barking commands just to establish that you can be bossy and loud. Your commands also help you discern a person's intent. Most of the commands you issue will be to establish and maintain—or regain—your bubble of safety.

According to police, if a person continues to move toward you after you've commanded him to stop, this is cause to consider this *a physical threat of a physical assault.* Following a plan also mentally places you in the here and now.

Take a lesson from professionals: law enforcement officers are gentle and polite (but always in command in any circumstance) until they need to be assertive and stern. Then they raise their intensity, stop giving instructions,

---

[65] "7 Memorable Quotes From Gen. James 'Mad Dog' Mattis" (accessed December 20, 2017); available from http://abcnews.go.com/Politics/memorable-quotes-gen-james-mad-dog-mattis/story?id=43693457

and start issuing commands and taking strong actions. Aside from respect for others and law and order, why do people not mess with a cop? Because they know there will be consequences. Deliberately projecting the image of a hard target by being overtly aware, issuing verbal commands (**Back off!**), and taking strong action puts predators on notice that you are not a meek victim looking for a place to be attacked.

Acting from power both depends on and projects *confidence.*

These steps move you from a weak position of merely reacting (victim) to acting (defender). Remember, if you wait to see what a Threat will do, you will see (and feel) what the Threat does. That is not a plan. Victims Vacillate; Defenders Decide.

Rehearsing your Five Step Plan (quietly in public and out loud at home) helps you turn your self-protection mindset into a habit.

* * *

The late heavyweight karate world champion Joe Lewis (not to be confused with heavyweight boxer Joe Louis) had some things to say about "street fighters" in an article he wrote for *Black Belt* magazine. Having won eleven national and world titles in a two-year period and having had his skills tested on the street, some people still consider him the greatest fighter ever. Here's his summation in that article:

"Lastly, I can assure you that a much greater number of ring fighters have tested and proven their skills in the 'street' than the number of street fighters who have ever entered the ring. If you took 10 top ring fighters and 10 top street fighters and let each group test their skills in the other's forum, which would have the higher winning percentage? A ring fighter's abilities will always, hands down, work far better for him in the street than a street fighter's abilities could ever help him in a ring fight."[66]

---

[66] "Exposing The Myth" (accessed May 5, 2016); available from http://www.bullshido.net/forums/showthread.php?t=96583

8

SEE AND AVOID THREATS

"Guys...awareness, awareness, awareness." — *Nick Drossos of Code Red Defense™*

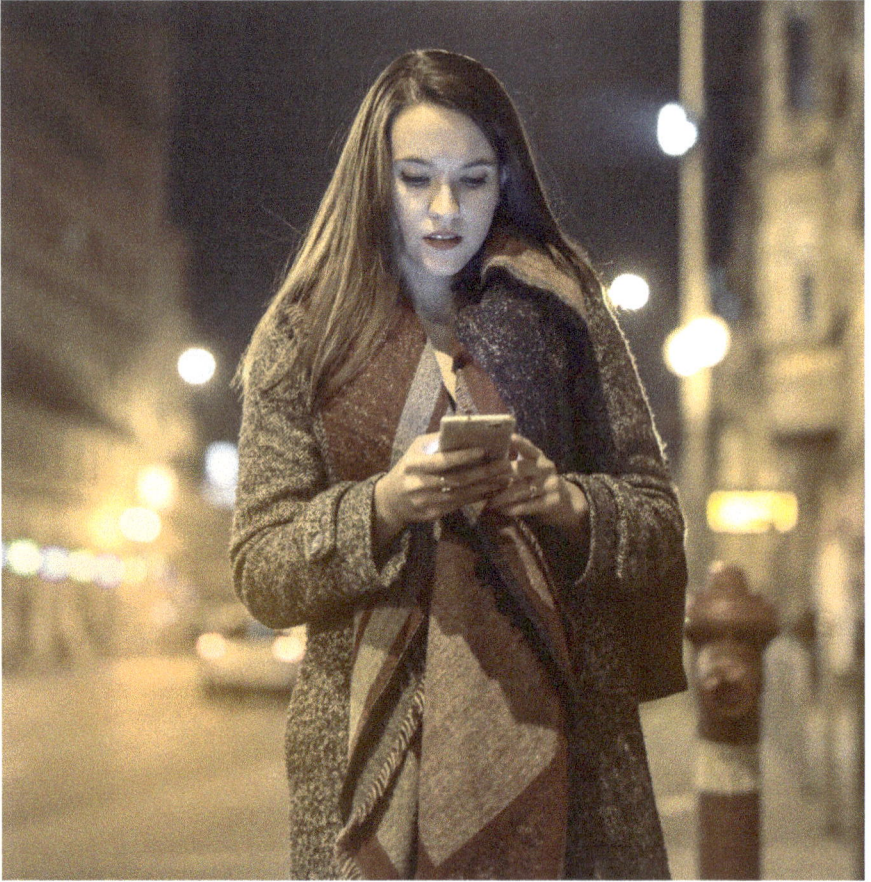

Walking alone at night, head down, with her focus of attention directed to her cell phone, is not part of our proactive Five Step plan. Photo: Andrea Piacquadio

When in Doubt, Chicken Out.

Awareness can provide time to flee, comply (robbery), or prepare for a violent confrontation. Whether you carve out time to physically train and practice fighting techniques or not, awareness is the keystone of self-protection.

The awareness steps I offer require little effort and no time. You can and should practice these easy skills as you move about during your normal routines until they are habit, without taking any time away from any of your other activities. I have placed a list of awareness and verbal avoidance drills in the Pulling It All Together chapter.

Physical "self-defense" (fighting) training teaches that to survive in a physical confrontation you must go and stay on offense. Think of our entire Five Step Plan as *being on offense: actively scanning, planning and executing.*

To stay aware of your surroundings and perceive any potential or actual **Threats,** think as Law Enforcement Officers (LEOs) do: **keep your head on a swivel.** Recall that when discussing human threats, they have the opportunity, ability, and intent to do you harm.

How often should you be scanning? Enough so you have ***complete knowledge of your environment and its threats and resources***. In many types of attacks, predators try to avoid being recognized as threats until they attack. If there is a predator nearby, he will try to be the one person you fail to notice or recognize as trouble. Fighter pilots say, "The airplane that shoots you down is the one you didn't see."

You also need to be aware of **resources** you can take advantage of—e.g., open businesses or crowds where you can get lost. Firefighters tell us that when indoors, we must **always know where the exits (safety) are**. For our purposes, we consider doors two-way exits: to get out of a building in case of fire or into a building to escape a parking lot predator, for instance. Try to always know "exits" in different directions. When you spot a potential Threat, you want to flee *to* safety not simply *away* from the Threat.

Keep it simple.

- **Keep your head on a swivel.**
- **Know two directions to flee to get to safety**.

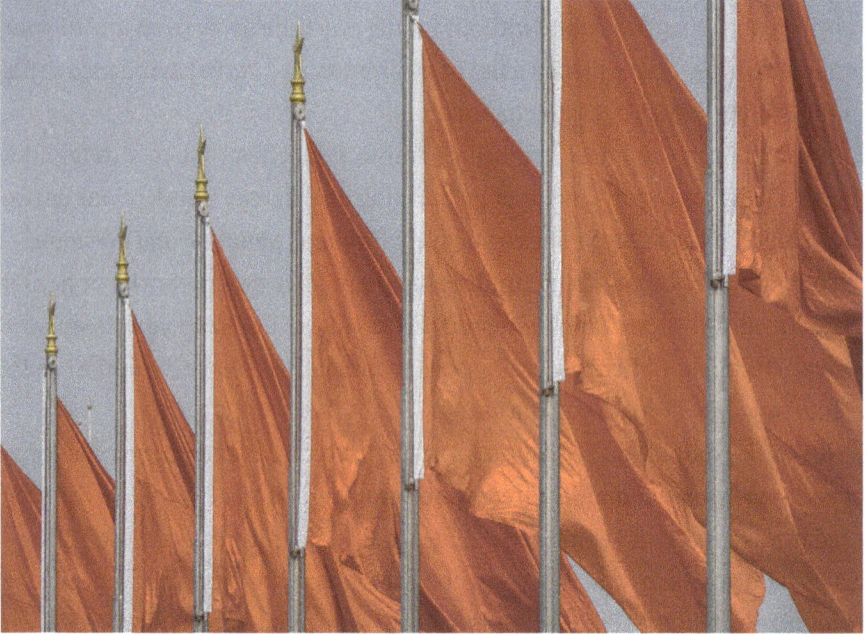

Photo: Mike Van Schoondervalt

Here are a few **Red Flags** that warn you when your awareness has not kept up with changes in your environment:

- **Fixation or Distraction:** you're focusing on something to the exclusion of all else. It might be important, or it could be an intentional distraction by a predator (more on this later).
- **Ambiguity:** is an uneasy state in which you're confused by conflicting cues and unsure of your safety. This can occur when your environment rapidly changes. Knowing high-threat environments helps you maintain proper alertness.
- You get **surprised** by something that should have been obvious.
- **Complacency:** you catch yourself unaware—and you are okay with it.
- **Fatigue** and effects of legal or illicit substances can make you more susceptible to any of these things.

One of the most important benefits of recurrent training in any job is shaking off whatever complacency has sneaked into the trainee's habits. These include flight crewmembers, train engineers, ship or boat operators and others in transportation, Law Enforcement Officers, EMTs, firefighters, vehicle maintenance technicians, military personnel and medical caregivers, heavy equipment operators, electricians, snowplow operators, as well as all the people who train them—the list goes on and on. These people's competence directly influences someone's well-being and safety. **Complacency kills**.

When discussing investments, financial advisers use the phrase, "Past performance does not guarantee future results." Just because you have walked across the dark parking lot at work dozens of times without incident *does not* mean trouble cannot find you. Criminals' schemes often depend on their targets' complacency.

Unfortunately, predators continue to refine their skills at finding brief instances when you are focusing your attention mostly on some task and less on your surroundings.

Scan: The eyes have it.

> *"Focus your mind, focus your eyes, focus your body."* —*Grandmaster Ralph Kreimer*

How do we best notice people to avoid? How can we at least be aware of people we can't avoid?

Let's recall how to best use our eyes.[67]

- Keeping your gaze on what you wish to see works best in bright light and lets you see details and colors; look right where you want to see.
- Your peripheral vision works is superior in dim light and better detects

---

[67] "How Your Eyes Work" (accessed January 13, 2016); available from http://www.aoa.org/patients-and-public/resources-for-teachers/how-your-eyes-work?sso=y

motion. This is why you often see something move "out of the corner" of your eye. If you want to examine something in low light, look slightly to the side of your subject, to better use your peripheral vision.

· In order to see motion, you have to hold your eyes steady. Search, stopping for a few moments in different directions—including behind you.

· Unfortunately, you are much better at noticing *relative motion* than changes in an object's apparent *size*. That means—unfortunately—a person who crosses your visual field (neither moving directly toward nor away from you) is easier to spot than a person who is coming straight at you because that second person's image merely appears to grow gradually larger; there is no relative movement. You are less likely to notice the person or moving object you most need to see.

Obviously, due to the speeds involved, pilots *constantly* need to keep their heads on swivels to stay aware of their environment including air traffic around them. Two airliners flying in exactly opposite directions, nose-to-nose, at cruise speed are getting five football fields closer to each other each second. Even light airplanes of the type you see flying around small airports will be closing head-to-head at nearly one football field per second. However, most mid-air collisions occur with the aircraft meeting at angles such that neither aircraft appears at the 12 o'clock position of the other. This is because an airplane, car, or person, approaching from any angle, that is on a collision course with you, will only appear to grow larger and is less noticeable if off to your side. An object or person moving across your field of vision will not intercept you (unless you or that other moving object changes course). Couple high closure rate with no apparent motion of the other airplane (it only appears to grow gradually larger) and you can see why pilots stay heads-up and scanning. *Pilots scan by looking methodically back and forth, pausing every 30 or so degrees*, looking for other airplanes near their altitude. Use the pilot's methodical scanning technique.

· Getting fully acclimated to seeing at night requires half an hour or more.

During World War II, US Navy sailors who stood watch on a ship's deck were required to spend thirty minutes in a low-light environment before going outside to begin a night watch.[68] A predator who has been lurking in the darkness for hours can see better than you can right after you move from a bright environment to a dim one. Look around as well as *listen*.

- You don't always notice things above or below your visual field. Pick up your cell phone and look at it while standing. Where are you holding it? Practice holding your phone at chin level so you can see over it. With your arm nearly straight, your peripheral vision is more available to spot movement. This also reminds you to look around.

- "Riding the front wheel" is an expression motorcycle racers use to describe the mistake of not looking far enough ahead. That gets racers into trouble—fast. When your head is on a swivel, it is important that you don't just focus on what's nearby in your little bubble. Expand that area by alternating your focus between close to you and further away, whether indoors or outdoors. Make this a habit.

- Remember from the video link in the Risk chapter: Benny "The Jet" Urquidez says proper posture aids good vision.[69] A proper or stealth fighting stance allows you to take in all of an enemy. Without moving your head or eyes, you should be able to observe the person's face and toes. (If you can't, he's probably too close to you.) In other words, use your vertical peripheral vision to notice any movement. By focusing on a person's eyes or just over his shoulder and holding your gaze still, **your peripheral vision will pick up movement faster than your focused vision.** At close range, a quarter of a second counts. This takes practice.

"The ears are the eyes of darkness." —*Grandmaster Ed Parker*[70]

---

[68] Discussion with the late US Navy Seaman First Class R.E. Lewis.

[69] "5 Rules of Discipline" (accessed January 8, 2018); available from http://bennythejet.com/5-rules-of-discipline.asp

[70] https://www.oocities.org/timmorrisonbelfast/wisdom/martial_arts.html

Don't forget your ears: hearing is your 360-degree early warning sense. Cockpits have many gauges and warning lights, yet for the most time-critical emergencies, warning bells or horns alert pilots to the danger, no matter where their eyes are focusing. This is the same concept as emergency responder vehicle sirens, your ears telling your eyes where to look.

By overtly keeping your head on a swivel you declare to predators: *I am not a soft target.* Projecting that you are a hard target is an avoidance tactic.

The Crux: Searching For Differences.

If you are focusing on everyone at once, you're really focusing on no one. As you move about, actively observe individual people or groups, starting from nearby and then outward. One way to ensure your observation is complete is to copy what lifeguards do: count people. That forces you to look around and individually observe each potential threat. When a pilot begins the exterior preflight inspection ("walk around") of an airplane, she first takes in the entire aircraft from a distance, then focuses on individual components when she's closer. If anything looks, sounds, or smells (overheating metal or leaking fluids) different, she gives it extra attention. Preflight the people near you.

Whenever I did the walk around of an airplane I was about to fly, I played a mental game. I assumed there was something wrong (different) with the airplane, and I had to find it—an Easter egg hunt. If I found a problem, I began the game again, so I'd keep searching. *Problems—and predators—are not always identified by sight*; a preflight inspection also means being alert for sounds that shouldn't be there, or should be but are not, and paying attention to whether there is an odor that shouldn't be there.

Speaking of odors, while you watch and listen, be alert for the characteristic smell of alcohol *consumption* on a person's breath.

[Side note: You notice that it doesn't smell like alcohol. That characteristic smell of drinking is once-oxidized ethyl alcohol (ethanol), which has become acetaldehyde. You can smell it because unlike ethanol, acetaldehyde is a gas at body temperature and passes from the blood to air via the lungs, where it is exhaled.]

Hear intentionally—especially for someone behind you. Then confirm what you hear by looking at the person behind you, thus announcing that you're aware and you take initiative.

Together with your life experience, the cues below may help you decide who you should actively observe or move away from.

It is important to watch out for: people whose body language conveys dominant behavior, people who look uncomfortable or hyper vigilant with their eyes darting in all directions or display the "thousand yard stare". Also be wary of people who are unfocused or unusually fixated and those who are loud, obnoxious, or uncommunicative when addressed. These behaviors do not guarantee that the people displaying them are threats, but they warrant further observing, so why not avoid them to reduce stress?

Group what you can sense about a person into categories:

- *Physical characteristics* as they pertain to their ability to harm (or help) you or run faster than you can (age, reach and weight, apparent fitness, agility—how he moves, whether his clothing will slow him down, etc.)
- The appearance *choices* of a person matters, so take those in as well. Is he wearing attire appropriate for your setting? Does he respect himself enough to practice good hygiene? These things may seem trivial, but they are clues as to who you are encountering.
- What is his *behavior*—both voluntary and involuntary? Does he appear to be impaired by mental illness or substances? Does he look nervous? Does he display calm or agitation? Is he paying abnormal attention to anyone in particular? Are his behavior and speech appropriate for the setting?
- Is he carrying any *weapons*? Can you see for certain that his hands (fingers) are empty? Are there bulges around his belt line or armpits? Is he wearing concealing, cold weather clothing on a warm day? What is he carrying? Police officers spot concealed firearms from yards away, and and are trained to instruct "Show me your hands" because hands kill.

- Does this person trigger your *gut feeling*? Look and listen for people who are not doing what everyone else is. That indicates they are not present for the same reasons as others.

A simple people-watching tip: wherever you are, ensure you have a good view of the people. Where applicable, pick a spot indoors near an entrance and exit point and from which you can see most of the people in your vicinity. Try to keep your back to a wall to avoid surprises.[71] If possible, have unimpeded access to an exit—and know where they are located—at all times. You don't want to be the last person in the room to figure out you should leave.

Detailed people observing works so well that a specific technique called Behavior Pattern Recognition has been used in "profiling [airline] passengers based not on race or religion but on suspicious and deceitful behavior".[72] It allows trained security personnel to reliably pick out bad actors by noticing *subconscious* little movements they make, which are *different* than how people normally move. Become a people observer. Search for people doing something abnormal—even a seemingly minor detail. If you decide they might be Threats, if you find them simply questionable, move away from them. **You do not have to be right; you just have to be careful.**

Certainly this gut feeling could cause you to avoid someone who turns out not to be a Threat. Perhaps someone is from another culture and this is why he or she is acting differently than you expect. Honor your instinct and unobtrusively move away without offending him or her.

You ladies know that a male stranger trying to engage you while apart from others, say in a parking lot or on an empty sidewalk or on an exercise or hiking trail, is out of place and will feel threatening. Know that we men are keenly

---

[71] "How to Develop the Situational Awareness of Jason Bourne" (accessed February 1, 2017), available from http://www.artofmanliness.com/2015/02/05/how-to-develop-the-situational-awareness-of-jason-bourne/. This webpage has a clip from one of the Bourne movies that shows hyper situational awareness, or SA.

[72] "Behavior Pattern Recognition and Aviation Security" (accessed November 10, 2023); available from https://www.tandfonline.com/doi/abs/10.1300/J460v01n02_06

aware of that, too, and we avoid making eye contact or approaching you in such circumstances. A male who violates this cultural no-no is *very* different and deserves a very wide berth. ***Rude Is The New Safe*** is your mantra.

Your safety is more important than courtesy or others' feelings. Protecting yourself *will* require you to be rude or even offensive at times. Always putting others' feelings above yours is called "people pleasing" and "chronic people pleasing equals chronic stress."[73]

Nick Drossos of *Code Red Defense*™ recommends you not limit your searching to finding bad actors, but also play a game of watching other people's security habits and mentally critiquing them. This can help sharpen your habits or find gaps in your awareness.

Precautions

The following bullet point reminders apply before you've decided an attack is imminent.

- Project the image of a hard target.
- When people pass you walking in the opposite direction (especially if they've greeted you), glance over your shoulder to see whether they've looked back at you or even turned around.
- Do not look at your phone while walking around. That marks you as a soft target.
- **Different Is A Red Flag**—a signal that something's wrong. Avoid people who are acting or presenting themselves differently than everyone else in your setting.
- Avoid or get away from drinking males (watch, listen, and smell for clues).
- Get away from anyone who keeps buying you drinks. Alcohol is a favored

---

[73] "Seven Ways People Chronic Pleasing Ruins Your Health" (accessed June 1, 2016); available from http://www.naturalnews.com/041439_people_pleasing_self-sabotage_self-confidence.html

weapon of sexual predators. If you turn your attention away from an uncovered drink, even momentarily, that drink is no longer yours. Put it down where you won't pick it up again.

· Get away from anyone who seems determined to get you alone.

· Never be alone with a male until he has *earned* your trust over considerable time.

· Stay with your group when returning to your cars. Drive each other to your cars or take a taxi if called for. Parking areas are common crime areas.

· Do remember that likely venues for violent crimes are residences, commercial places and schools (through high school); and for property crimes the highest-risk locations are in or near home and parking areas.

Real Life People Observing

I had just landed an Airbus 320, finishing a trip at Washington Reagan Airport late one warm summer night. While walking across the skybridge that connects the terminal to a public parking garage, I found myself in the company of two males in their twenties. They wore shorts and T-shirts. Nothing in their hands. They walked the same curiously slow speed, several feet apart and not talking to one another. The men were too far apart to look like they were together, yet too close to each other to be walking separately in the nearly vacant passageway. Even though I was tired, my head stayed on a swivel: their **different** (**Red Flag**) pace and interval marked them as possible Threats and the three of us were walking toward a (increased-risk) parking area.

Walking ahead of them I stopped at one of the parking pay machines located just short of the garage. Turning to face them I freed my hands by setting my bag between me and their approach. I could see them inching toward me while I paid. They each scrutinized me as they closed in. I observed three exit paths open to me.

They skipped the pay machines and walked past me into the garage. I saw them turn and stroll along the perimeter of the structure, away from the parked cars.

We know that **Different Is A Red Flag**. You've already picked out some things they were doing differently than other people in this late-night airport context.

- They weren't dressed or badged as airport employees, and they were leaving the terminal of an airport late at in the evening—this most likely meant they had just arrived on a flight. But, people who've arrived on a flight and are exiting the terminal always have things in their hands. They appeared to be neither employees nor passengers.
- Late at night, leaving an airport, most people are high-tailing it to their cars, eager to get home. These two weren't.
- Their strange spacing served the purpose of a head start to approach a victim from two directions.
- Since they didn't use a pay machine they likely didn't have a car in that garage: What were they doing there?
- Each made extensive and challenging eye contact with me, which was a further indication that they were together and no strangers to trouble.
- They didn't walk toward the cars in the garage.

How many of these cues would I have missed had I been reading text messages or talking on my phone instead of keeping my head on task?

My car was on a higher level, so I took the elevator up and never saw them again.

Gut check: What would you have done—and when—in that situation?

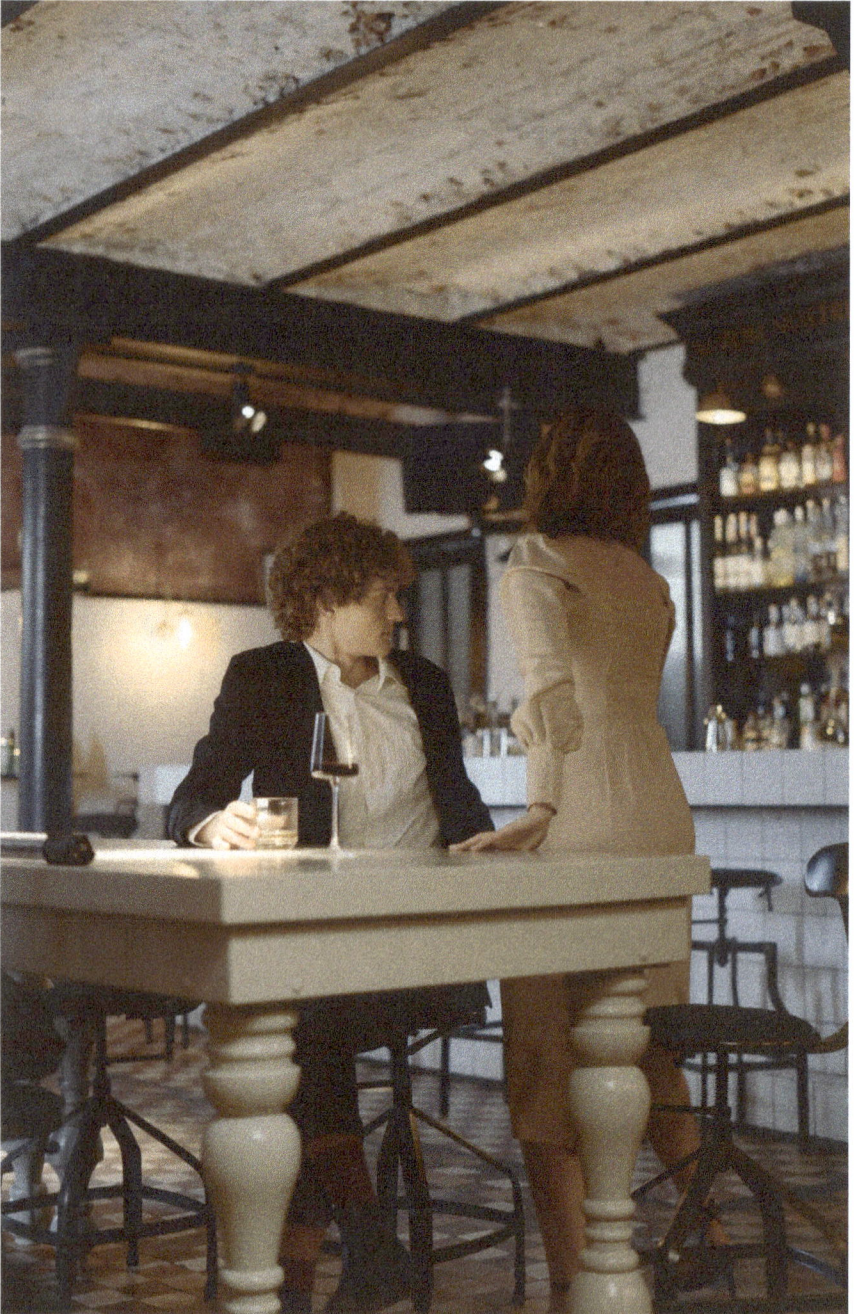

Unless this woman trusts this man with her life, that drink she's turned her back on is no longer safe. Photo: Cottonbro Studio

Help

It makes sense to have close, long-term, trustworthy friends or family around when you're in remote locations, out late at night or in other areas where a Threat can be lurking: exercise paths, parking areas, streets, and at parties even in private places.

If your work begins or ends in darkness, plan to have a trusted person or two to walk you between your car and your employer's building. Predator fish don't attack schools of smaller fish. They isolate and zero in on one particular fish. Staying in schools makes fish much harder to prey upon. Human predators do the same: *isolate and attack.* Do not isolate yourself for them.

Sit-down restaurants have people standing just inside their doors—as do hotels, which often also have their own security guard. Bars have big guys who work the door. Eateries, hotels, and pubs are usually open late. If you're concerned about your safety, walk in and ask for help. Remain there until you are certain that leaving is safe. If prudent, call someone to pick you up where you are.

Police do not hesitate to call for assistance when they need it, and they're armed, trained and experienced. In fact, they have rules directing them to have a sufficient number of officers present in various situations. Plan or enlist help.

Remember: having help available to you doesn't mean only while you're out jogging or shopping. It also means you're not alone with males who haven't yet earned your trust—whether in residences, vehicles, or anywhere else. Before going on dates alone with a guy, make him earn your trust by spending time with him in places where the two of you won't be isolated—including where your parents or friends can put more eyes on him.

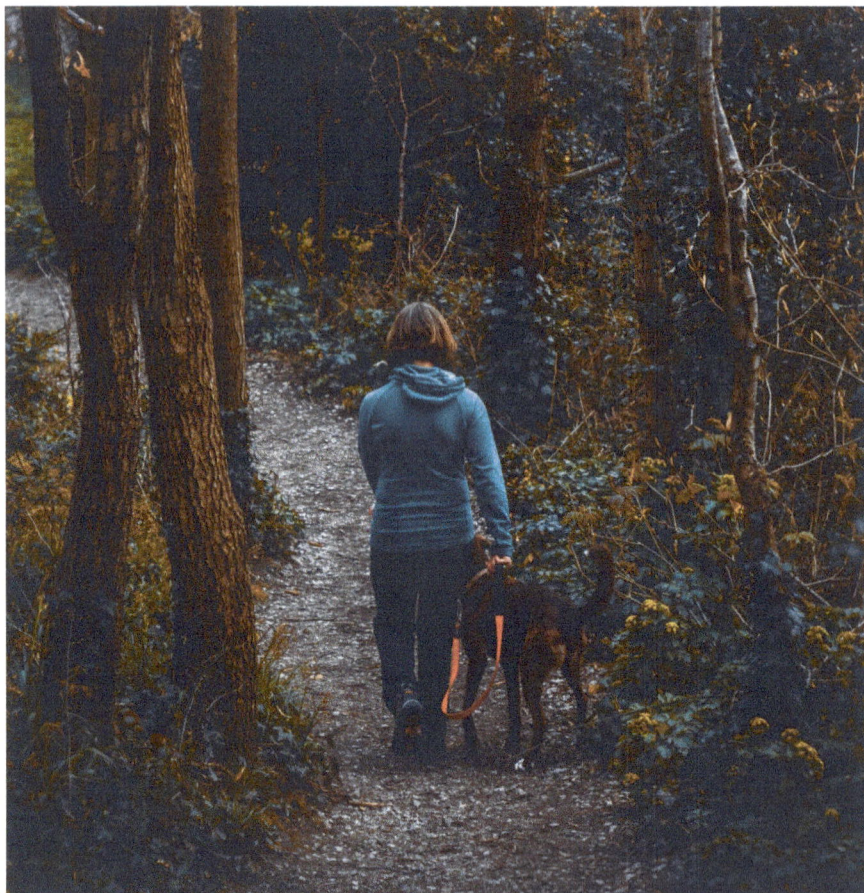

This woman has a good helper with her. Photo: Lisa Fotios

* * *

Since the first time two aircraft were airborne simultaneously, "see and avoid" has been the primary way airplanes flying in clear air avoid colliding. *See and avoid is a survival skill.* This very good three-minute video shows you how to be—and look—aware as you move about. *See and avoid.* Click HERE.[74]

---

[74] "True Awareness In Self Defense" (accessed May 18, 2021); available from https://www.yout ube.com/watch?v=NR6Q3Ujzicc

9

EVERYONE IS NOT "JUST LIKE ME."

"Violence, naked force, has settled more issues in history than has any other factor; and the contrary opinion is wishful thinking at its worst. Breeds that forget this basic truth have always paid for it with their lives and their freedoms."[75]
—*Robert A. Heinlein's character Jean V. Debois* (Starship Troopers)

---

[75] Heinlein, Robert A., "Starship Troopers," (New York: Berkley, 2018)

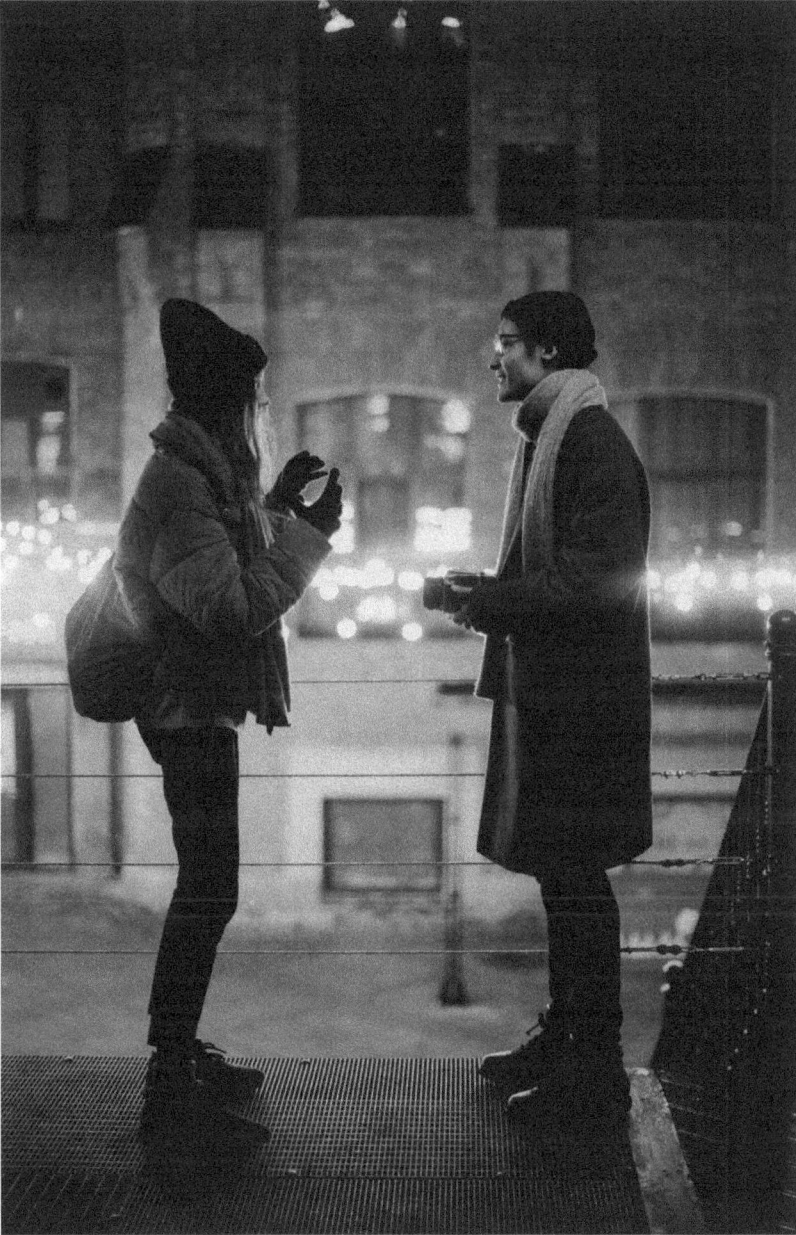

*Is anyone walking up behind her? When you stop for a stranger, you make yourself a stationary target. By engaging in conversation you lose awareness of your surroundings. **Rude Is The New Safe**: It's usually safer to keep moving.*
Photo: Cottonbro Studio

K

now Your Enemy, Know Yourself

Knowing yourself and your enemy was advice given in *Art of War*, by Sun Tzu.[76]

Our Enemy:

Believes he has the right to prey

Angered by those who thwart him

Deals with others via confrontation and conquest

Seeks and recognizes soft targets

Uses overwhelming, needless violence

Manipulates conditions of attack for his advantage

Experienced at attacking

Acts to surprise us

Can break off attack at will

Distracts with conversation

Ourselves:

---

[76] *Sun Tzu on the Art of War*, Sun Tzu (public domain translation by Lionel Giles, M.A., 1910); written circa 500 BC. This book is still studied by our military.

"Everyone is just like me."

Live and let live.

Deal with others by communication and cooperation

May project that we are a soft target

Expect life to be fair much of the time

May be unaware of our disadvantages

Not experienced at fighting back

Predators often catch us by surprise

Our defense has to be 100% effective

Hesitate to prioritize our safety over others' wants and feelings

Are you mentally prepared to respond to an encounter with a brutal predator? We read news stories of gruesome violence and ask ourselves why the criminal chose to inflict needless harm. The fact is, the predator has crazy reasons that seem rational to him. Repeat this until you believe it: "**Everyone is *not* just like me.**"

Deception

"All warfare is deception." —*Sun Tzu*

A man stowed the groceries he'd just purchased into his car. It was mid-day at a crowded shopping center. With cars moving in the aisles he had chosen to stand between his car and another vehicle and load through the side door into the back

seat instead of utilizing the trunk. A man approached him in the narrow space. The stranger asked him for directions to the city library. A moment later, a second stranger—unseen and unheard by the man—struck the victim from behind and then again in the face, breaking his jaw. Down the man went. The thugs grabbed his wallet and ran; the victim was semiconscious, unsure of what had happened to him. This brutal attack took place in the middle of the day with people milling about and a busy, four-lane street right next to the full parking lot. It shouldn't happen in those conditions, right?

This was the day of the month when social security checks get deposited—and retirees withdraw cash and go shopping. Predators know how, when, and where to prey.

Notice the man wasn't given the chance to turn over his wallet and avoid the beating—the crooks didn't want to take the time or risk him making noise. This is typical of robberies by unarmed assailants. No mercy. The violence was over in two seconds; the entire incident in 10 seconds. No do-overs. Your awareness and defense have to be right, every time.

What could the victim have done better?

- He was trapped between cars (what Sun Tzu called "entrapping ter-rain"—where no army wants to be). He could have loaded the groceries into the trunk instead of through one of the doors. Most fighters will tell you that if attacked, they want room to run away or at least move around—especially if confronted with multiple or armed attackers. **Train yourself to think tactically.** Look at everyday tasks and situations from the perspectives of a defender *and* an attacker. As Yogi Berra noted, "You can observe a lot just by watching."
- The victim lost focus on his surroundings; he didn't see either thug approaching.
- He trusted someone he'd never met and allowed the stranger to hijack his attention.
- The victim didn't keep his head on a swivel. Looking around is extra

important when you could be trapped. Awareness can buy you time to escape.

As we've noted, victims of violent crimes are often shocked and wonder how someone they have never offended—or even met—could attack them so savagely. There are thugs who would do the same to us without hesitation or remorse.

Note how the thugs preyed on our natural inclination to help others. The more helpful we can be, the better we feel, and feelings are powerful. *Eagerly helping to the exclusion of healthy cynicism is volunteering to be a victim. Staying focused on our safety requires relentless discipline formed by constant practice, which is entirely up to you.*

"Focus, Daniel-san!"[77]

You have two types of attention: focus of attention and margin of attention.

Your margin of attention allows you to do routine tasks, seemingly without thinking about them (such as walking).

For complex tasks you must use your focused attention. Magicians and predators know these things: they direct your gaze away from what they are really doing, and that lets them surprise you. Magicians call this *misdirection*. During Athena Women training, and in the Pulling It All Together chapter, we present scenarios involving this tactic.

---

[77] The character Mr. Miagi, played by the late Noriyuki "Pat" Morita, *The Karate Kid*, Columbia Pictures Corporation, 1984. If you haven't yet seen it, do so.

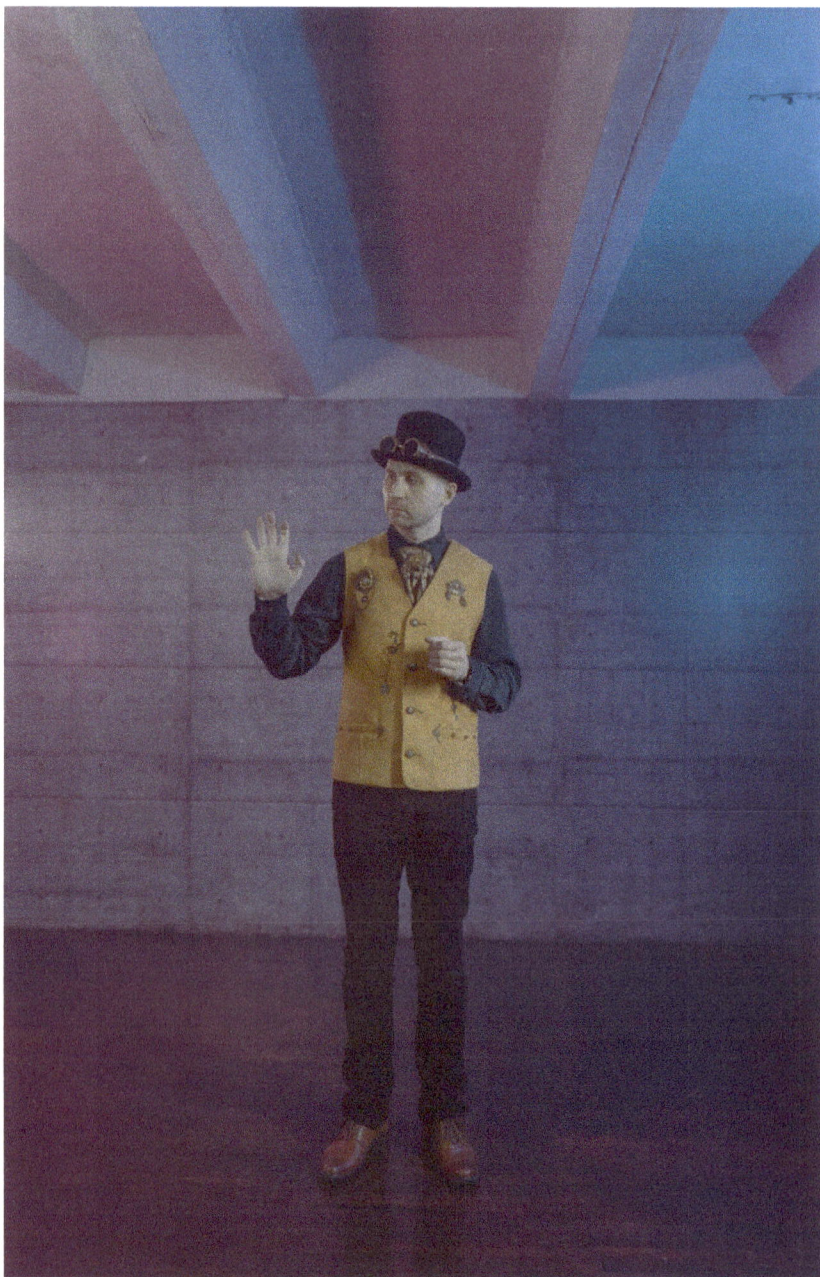

Quick: Which of this magician's hands did you look at first? Which hand could be holding a weapon? His open hand and where he is looking both worked to misdirect your attention. Photo: Tima Miroshnichenko

You are a single channel being, meaning **you can only focus on one thing at a time.** Today, computer work terminals in an office or school are stand-alone computers hooked together. However, when computers were just becoming common, those work terminals weren't actually computers because computers were too large to fit on top of desks. Those terminals were connected to one large, main computer that did all the processing. That main computer could only "pay attention" to one terminal at a time. That way of functioning was called time-sharing.

In the same way, your brain focuses on each task *one at a time.* Each activity gets *all* of your brain's focus of attention for a while, and then your focus shifts to another task for a time, and so on. When you think you are multi-tasking, you are instead rapidly alternating your attention between tasks (time-sharing) and you may not notice you are performing each of them less proficiently. This is why it *is* impossible for you to text and drive at the same time—every moment you are either texting *or* driving, never both. In fact, safety-first Volvo believes that up to 90% of all traffic accidents are caused by drivers whose focus of attention wandered toward something other than driving.[78]

The most important rule pilots must follow when handling an inflight emergency is "someone must fly the airplane." One pilot must keep her focus of attention on flying at all times while the other pilot focuses his attention on the emergency. The most dangerous thing the flying pilot can do is to try to "help" the non-flying pilot deal with the emergency. The flying pilot ends up doing both poorly because there is no such thing as multi-tasking. The lives of the pilots, their crew, and passengers depend on a the flying pilot's ability to focus on one thing only: flying the airplane. In fact, FAA regulations forbid airline pilots from even talking about anything non-operational when maneuvering below 10,000 feet above Mean Sea Level (MSL). The aviation community has known for decades that *where we focus our attention can mean*

---

[78] "City Safety by Volvo Cars – outstanding crash prevention that is standard in the all-new XC90" quoting If Insurance Company of Sweden (accessed May 31, 2016); https://www.m edia.volvocars.com/global/en-gb/media/pressreleases/154717/city-safety-by-volvo-cars-outstanding-crash-prevention-that-is-standard-in-the-all-new-xc90

STAYING SAFE FOR TODAY'S WOMAN

the difference between life and death.

That only-one-thing-at-a-time limitation on your focus of attention is important to you for two reasons.

First, if you pay attention to anything besides your environment, then you cannot be focusing on what's happening around you. When your head stops swiveling, that's what we call a clue: you may have lost awareness.

Second, the criminal tries to force you to pay attention to the cues *he wants* you to focus on—to make you miss what's really going on. He doesn't want you to notice him or his maneuvers (such as placing himself in perfect distance and angle to knock you down with a sucker punch or getting an accomplice to approach you from behind). In cyber terms, the criminal is the equivalent of the internet pop-up ad that steals your attention for at least a moment. He prevents you from quickly responding to the attack when it *seems to you* to occur suddenly. In reality, **the attack began as soon as you let the stranger engage you in conversation.** Reread that.

When a potential Threat penetrates your bubble, one of the most important things to look for is what their hands are doing: check for weapons and whether he is positioning his hands to strike you.

Notice that head *swiveling* and *fixation* are mutually exclusive.

The good news is that **you choose where you center your attention**. To develop good attention habits you absolutely must practice being intentional about this.

· Everyone around you falls into one of three categories: trusted, not trusted, and suspected Threat. **Trusted** is reserved for those who have *earned your trust over time*. Uniforms are the exception that proves this rule. Pilots, flight attendants, LEOs, security guards, fire fighters, doctors and nurses, and EMTs wear uniforms to tell you they're instantly trustworthy—this is necessary during emergencies. If your default operating mode is trusting everyone you meet (Puppy Dog Mode), you need to shift your thinking to consider strangers and recent acquaintances as **Not Trusted, or Not Yet Trusted**. The category of **Suspected Threat** is for someone who does something different (e.g., raises a **Red Flag**) or otherwise causes you to believe he may be dangerous. You do this naturally; try using this skill deliberately.

- Surprises (fast and s-l-o-w). You can be surprised by the sudden, violent attack of a stranger, or equally shocked by the gradual encroachment attack (employing verbal pressure, alcohol, persistence and perhaps eventually force) of someone you know.

No Rules

The captain of an airliner is responsible for everything that happens on her plane. She has unlimited authority to break all the rules, to **do whatever it takes** to land safely. You, too, can violate rules in order to be safe.

You do not live to please other people. Their problems are not yours to solve, and **rude and safe beats polite and assaulted**. You are not on a stranger's schedule, so do not let anyone rush you into making poor decisions. *You are not responsible for a stranger's hurt feelings.*

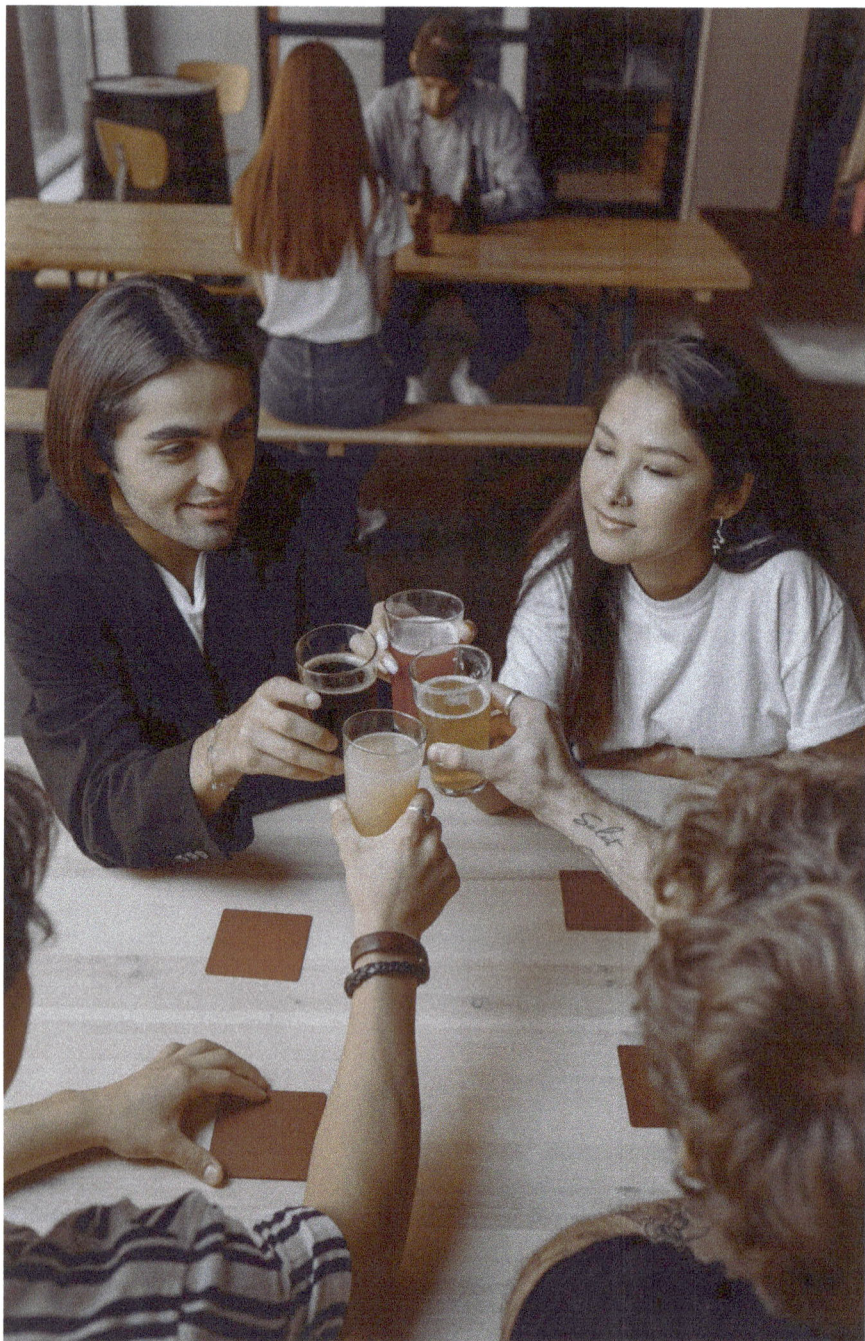

Remember: Everyone is NOT just like you. Photo: Cottonbro Studio

* * *

A thug jumped a 25-year-old woman who was a karate black belt and placed fourth in the Junior World Championships in 2007.

"I hit him in the ribs with my knee and punched him in the face as hard as I could... I think I broke his nose," said Taela Davis, of Skye, Australia, near Melbourne.

However, he kept fighting (he may have been drug-affected).

"I knew then that I'd have to beat the crap out of him," she said.

Fortunately for the attacker, a passerby came along, and the thug fled before that beating took place.[79]

If you haven't already, spend a few minutes deciding what you're willing to do to ensure you are prepared to fight back. ***This decision will possibly be the most important you will make regarding your personal safety.***

---

[79] "Thug assaults woman, but gets more than he bargained for when she turns out to be karate expert" (accessed May 6, 2016); available from http://www.heraldsun.com.au/leader/south-east/thug-assaults-woman-but-gets-more-than-he-bargained-for-when-she-turns-out-to-be-karate-expert/news-story/f30f28e3c819391fac550c06993aba72?nk=0f774adafefef930914470da3dd26bc6-1462563171

10

CONSENT OR COERCION?

"[you] are entitled to freedom of person..." —*Thomas Jefferson*

J ust because you know someone doesn't mean he will not attack you. Sexual predators' tools include physical force, getting you intoxicated or drugged, and verbal coercion. Strangers are more likely to use force while people you know usually use verbal coercion. Either can employ chemicals.

CONSENT: *"In the context of rape, submission due to apprehension or terror is not real consent. There must be a choice between resistance and acquiescence. If a woman resists to the point where additional resistance would be futile or until her resistance is forcibly overcome, submission thereafter is not consent."* [80]

Your "no" does not mean "yes".

Your silence does not mean yes.

Not fighting back does not mean yes.

---

[80] consent. (n.d.) A Law Dictionary, Adapted to the Constitution and Laws of the United States. By John Bouvier.. (1856). Retrieved December 14 2015 from http://legal-dictionary.thefreed ictionary.com/consent

Your fear does not mean yes.

COERCION: *"The intimidation of a victim to compel the individual to do some act against his or her will by the use of psychological pressure, physical force, or threats. The crime of intentionally and unlawfully restraining another's freedom by threatening to commit a crime, accusing the victim of a crime, disclosing any secret that would seriously impair the victim's reputation in the community..."*[81]

Any threat of violence or other, nonviolent, undesired consequence to you is coercion.

Verbally pressuring you is coercion.

Getting you drunk or drugged is coercion.

* * *

If you don't exercise command over your body, someone else will.

A command from you to a Threat, (*"Back off!,"* *"Stop!,"* *"No!"*) is not the first line in a conversation—it is the last.

* * *

---

[81] coercion. (n.d.) A Law Dictionary, Adapted to the Constitution and Laws of the United States. By John Bouvier.. (1856). Retrieved December 14 2015 from http://legal-dictionary.thefreed ictionary.com/coercion

Watch a Kathy Long kickboxing fight or highlights video online, such as THIS ONE. She's always on offense, *always taking the fight to her opponent.* (In a fight against a lone, unarmed attacker it is generally better to be moving forward than backward.) If you're ever forced to fight back physically *when you fear for your life*, you want to fight as she does until the danger has passed.

11

PULLING IT ALL TOGETHER: USING OUR FIVE STEP PLAN

"If you don't have a strategy you are part of someone else's strategy." —*Alvin Toffler*

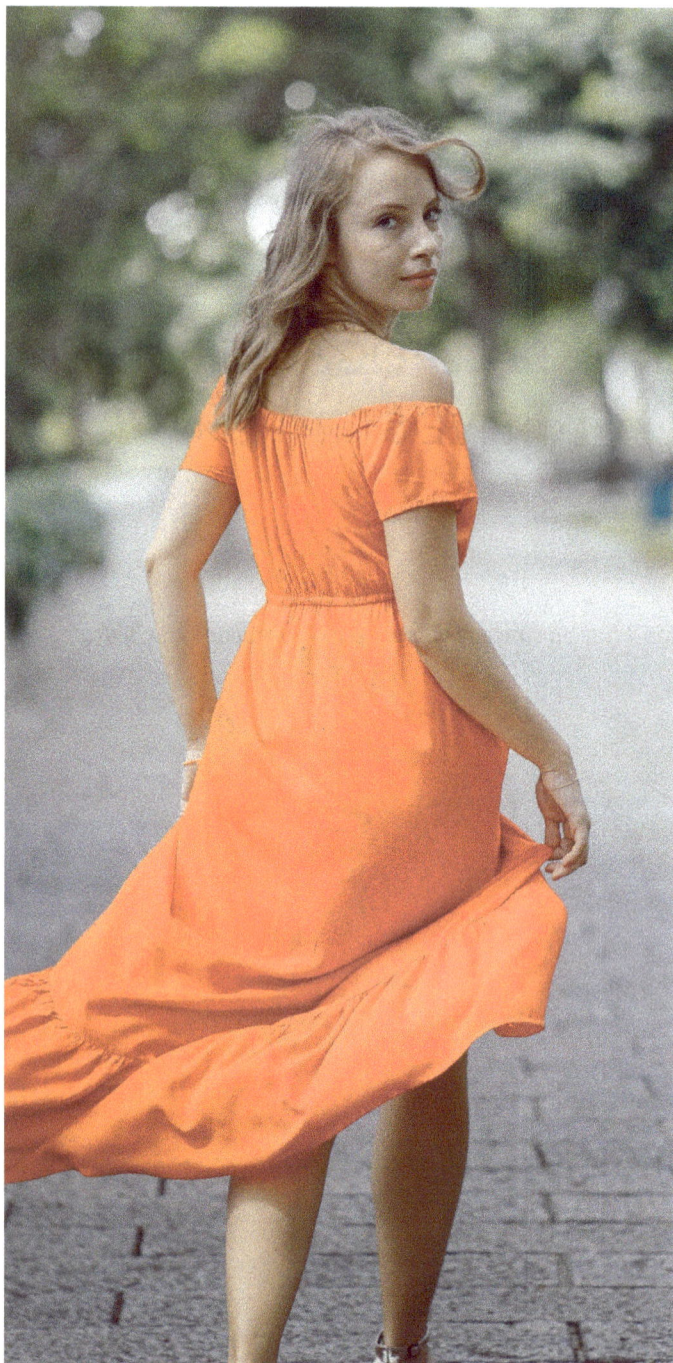

Good awareness—"checking her six" (o'clock). Photo: mentatdgt

Be Ready

At one point in my aviation career, I trained as an aircraft accident investigator. Investigators are always asked, "When did the accident begin?"

The incident might have begun with a windshear just moments before, or years prior when a piece of metal developed a small crack that grew over time. *When does an attack begin?* For example, when did the trouble begin for the three young women leaving the movie theater in the opening short story?

An assault could start long before you see the attacker. It might be put in motion when you make a decision to go for a run in the local park by yourself before sunrise or allow yourself to be alone in a dwelling, car, or remote area with a male who hasn't yet earned your trust. It could begin with you drinking an open beverage handed to you by the wrong guy. Maybe when someone turns around to follow you and you forget to "check your six" or you walk into a parking garage where an unseen thug awaits his next victim. It might begin when a male you know slowly violates your limits.

The point is, *an attack can be initiated without your immediate knowledge.* Remember your new awareness and avoidance skills.

From the See & Avoid Threats section:

- **Keep your head on a swivel.**
- **Be aware of at least two directions you can move in to flee to safety**.

Four Feet vs. Twenty-one Feet

From tests performed in 1983 by Lt. John Tueller, a firearms instructor with the Salt Lake City Police Department, twenty-one feet is the minimum distance separating an individual and officer, from which an officer is able to discern whether the person is a Threat, decide whether or not to react, draw a handgun from a holster, point toward the target (unsighted), and squeeze the trigger before the Threat can harm the officer.[82]

Anyone trained in carrying a handgun knows this number like her birthday because it is often quoted. Twenty-one feet represents **one and a half seconds away from you** for a person on a flat surface. Right now, look at something located at about that distance. An agile person at that spot can reach you in only a second and a half. I think we'd all like at least that much time to react to a violent attack, but even this is unlikely.

Four feet is the minimum American culture's social circle radius for strangers, and that happens to be just over an arm's reach for a six-foot tall person. Except in crowded, confined or accepted conditions—such as in an elevator or passing on a sidewalk—no stranger should move within this radius from you without your concurrence.

Some police use five feet, telling people who might be Threats to "give me five." Since people won't give you a twenty-one foot bubble, you should enforce at minimum the four feet our societal standards grant us. Where possible, reasonably expand your bubble according to your comfort zone. A person who busts through your bubble when instructed not to is raising a **Red Flag. Furthermore, according to police you may consider a person who refuses to honor your instruction to *BACK OFF!* and keeps moving toward you to be a Threat who is physically threatening you with a physical assault.**

What can you do if this happens?

Your Safety Or Even Your Life May Depend On Working Your Plan

Hick's Law tells us that the more alternatives we have, the more time we need to reach a decision.[83] When dealing with emergencies during which split seconds count, aviation and law enforcement procedures are streamlined and simplified. Depending on the context of the situation, think of a breach of

---

[82] "Revisiting the '21-Foot Rule'" (accessed May 13, 2018); available from http://www.policem ag.com/channel/weapons/articles/2014/09/revisiting-the-21-foot-rule.aspx

[83] Chrysoula Malogianni, "Hick's Law," (accessed May 1, 2016); available from https://msu.edu/ ~malogian/hickslaw.html

your personal bubble by someone you've commanded to stop as a potential emergency. You need to be ready to react with **"if-then"decision-making and physical steps** that you've drilled into your memory via **many repetitions**.

Practicing your awareness and avoidance skills during your normal routines takes little or no extra time and is necessary to make them a habit.

"With repetition comes knowledge." — *Erica Blitz of* Namaste Yoga

Keep your head on a swivel, move to safety, Flee or Comply if those actions can keep you safe, and *last of all*, fight. Recall that your goal is to *escape unharmed*. During an attack, your goal is not to fight to win, but fight to escape.

- **Aware:** imitate the police by keeping your head on a swivel.
- **Avoid/de-escalate:** Know safe directions you can use as escape routes. De-escalate by not getting drawn into dialog with a stranger. Toss your valuables if you believe you are accosted by a robber.
- **Flee:** once there is an opening to do so safely. If this isn't possible, move to the next step.
- **Comply:** means give up your valuables (if you haven't yet); comply does **NOT** mean submitting to an assault and **NEVER** means allowing an assailant to relocate you.
- **(Counter)Attack:** if none of the above tactics prevents an attacker from **physically assaulting you, counterattack. If the attacker is physically threatening you with a physical assault and you have no other options**, you can initiate a preemptive counterattack. Do so per the use-of-force criteria in your locale. The point of this book is to help you to never get to this step. To learn more about how to select training to fight back, see the Training Tips chapter.

In keeping with Grandmaster Joe Lewis's wisdom that planning ends with the first hit, *the actions of a predator may cut short or re-order this Five Step Plan.*

If an attacker suddenly gets close to you before you are aware of him, you may have to start at Flee, Comply or even Counterattack. On the other hand, if he only verbally intimidates you in the absence of any physical threats or actions, you'll have to refrain from using force. Even if you can de-escalate a confrontation with a suspected Threat, move away as soon as you can.

De-escalate And Escape Early—While You Can

If you feel the need to remove yourself from a situation *before violence starts*:

- Do not argue with people you do not know.
- Do not stop to converse with them either. When you stop you become a stationary target who has also lost awareness—known as *Victim Mode*.
- Be polite, respectful and agreeable but do not pander.
- Blame the timing of your exit on someone not present.
- Move away using de-escalation body language, such as palms up in front of you. Having your hands between you and a potential Threat also readies you for defensive or offensive violence.

Observing means perceiving with *all* your senses.

Sexual attacks and domestic violence are the most common types of assaults against women.[84] Sexual predators commonly use just enough compliance violence to accomplish their goal.

Unarmed robbers use sudden, devastating violence to disable male and female victims quickly, cutting short any attention-attracting arguing or scuffles. Armed robbers brandish weapons to scare their victims into complying.

---

[84] "Statistics" (accessed January 5, 2018); available from https://centerforfamilyjustice.org/community-education/statistics/ (Domestic violence includes sexual, physical, emotional, psychological and economic abuse.)

Despite the difference in the intensity of violence, in both sexual attacks and unarmed robberies it serves as a tool.

During a robbery, a de-escalation technique is to *immediately comply* by turning over your valuables before the thug is within arm's reach. You can practice doing this in the scenario exercises just ahead. There are right and wrong ways to toss your valuables.

As far as de-escalating a sexual attack, "Verbal de-escalation is ineffective with a predator" and, "Bargaining and pleading will probably backfire, simply increasing the Threat's sense of excitement."[85] You must act early to get away from anyone who triggers your *gut reflex*.

According to police, most domestic violence physical attacks do not spontaneously erupt; the violence is usually preceded by a verbal conflict. Leaving *quietly* may be the best way to de-escalate a worsening domestic dispute.

Flee

The farther away you see a potential Threat and make the decision to avoid him, the better chance you have of *safely* fleeing. This may mean sprinting out of a parking garage, or simply stepping into an open business. Safely fleeing means the Threat won't take a few steps and tackle you from behind.

Comply

If a thug is close enough, you can try throwing down your valuables near him but off to the side to get his attention, which will give you a few more seconds head start or even satisfy the thief enough that he grabs your things and leaves in search of his next victim. Thieves do not want fights, they want your stuff. Throwing your valuables off to the predator's side forces him to visibly make a decision about his priorities: you or your belongings. If you toss your valuables straight toward him on a line between the two of you,

---

[85] Rory Miller, *Facing Violence*, (Wolfeboro: YMAA Publication Center, 2011), 64. If you're curious about the propensity for violence of different types of criminals, I recommend this book.

his next action won't tell you anything about his intention until he gets to your tossed items. Unfortunately, too often unarmed muggers don't make demands before they launch their physical attack, so compliance may require fast action on your part, anticipating what he wants while he is still out of arm's reach. Reminder: complying does *not* mean yield to a sexual assault or allow yourself to be taken to a deadly second crime scene.

(Counter)Attack

This book doesn't try to teach you fighting skills; this discussion presents an overview to give you a few basic ideas about fighting and dispel some myths so you can make an informed decision about whether to train. **If you want to learn how to fight back, seek training, which should include training on determining exactly why and when and how to start fighting (within your local laws) and especially when to NOT use force.** For you trained fighters, knowing *how* to fight is of less use without also correctly and confidently discerning *at what moment* fighting is called for—and is *not* called for. This requires judgment that comes from knowledge of local laws and practicing scenarios. *I cannot overstate the importance of this point.* Start fighting too late and get seriously injured; begin before it's called for and go to jail for assault.

Unlike some sports, during a physical confrontation you cannot prevail by playing defense. If you have no choice but to physically engage a predator, protect yourself and switch to offense. Ideally, your protection technique also initiates your counterattack, as our sucker punch counter does. This is called *defensive offense and recall that this must remain within the reasonable force rule and you must cease using force when the danger has passed.* As early as possible, safely flee (which is what you wanted to do in the first place).

Is there a tactical (vs. legal) difference between fighting back and self-defense? The innovative martial arts legend Bruce Lee wrote about the subject and is said to have remarked that there is no such thing as self-defense, only what he called *defensive offense*.[86] **In other words, you defend (protect) yourself by going on offense** (you've probably heard the old saw that the best defense is a strong offense). When you are being physically assaulted, limiting yourself to only covering up in a defensive position doesn't force an attacker to stop. As long as he keeps striking or grappling with you, you will suffer increasing injuries and be less and less able to get away or protect yourself. Physically fighting back—using fighting techniques—is what Lee meant by "defensive offense". Force the attacker to make defending himself *his* immediate problem. And stop when the danger has passed.

The late former FBI agent G. Gordon Liddy said in his autobiography, *Will*, that he didn't worry about his enemies; he preferred his enemies worry about him.[87] Ponder right now the power in that outlook and the decisions it drives. A good start is projecting the image of a hard target to make an attacker worry about you.

You may be thinking, "I'm not ferocious…I know I need to learn how to fight back, but I'm still not sure I can."

Lie to yourself—and this applies to our entire Five Step Plan. According to motivational speaker and black belt Tom Muzila, your subconscious can't tell truth from fiction. It's naïve. It will believe whatever you tell it and then either hinder you or stay out of your way. This is why talking down to yourself is so damaging. Pump yourself up. *Really* pump yourself up: instead of telling yourself *I can fight back and escape* tell yourself *I've already fought, prevailed and escaped.* Keep telling yourself that and you will see your attitude come around and support your training instead of sabotage your training.[88]

Jiu jitsu (an art focused on ground fighting) practitioners say, *If you can't execute a technique, you're either doing the wrong technique or doing the technique wrong.* In Jiu jitsu, a more skilled but smaller practitioner can defeat an opponent of nearly twice his size and strength, as Royce Gracie did on

---

[86] John Little, ed., *Bruce Lee: Jeet Kune Do. Bruce Lee's Commentaries On The Martial Way.* North Clarendon: Charles E. Tuttle Co., Inc., 1997

[87] Liddy, G. Gordon, *Will.* (New York: St Martin's Press, 1980)

[88] "Major Attitude," *Martial Art*, March 2003, 66.

his way to his second UFC World Championship. Effective techniques avoid engaging in a contest of strength or size against a bigger attacker. How? Often by focusing the greatest possible amount of mass and strength of your body against a vulnerable part of the attacker's body. This concept also applies to striking arts such as karate or tae kwon do: applying your body's *weapons* against an attacker's vulnerable *targets*.

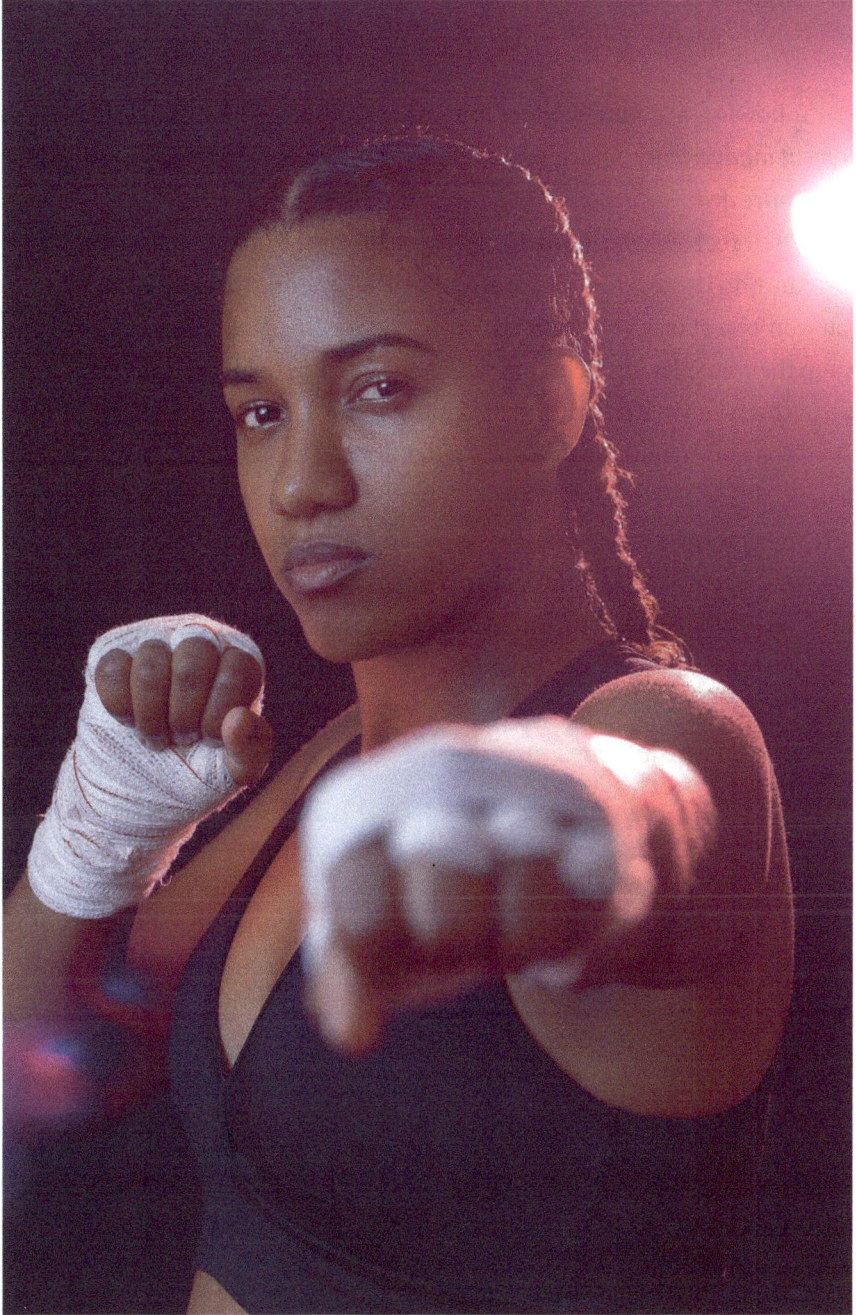

Even without the wrist wraps she broadcasts the image of a hard target. Photo: Ric Rodrigues

Awareness And Avoidance Training Scenarios

The following are **non-contact** scenarios we use during our training. *To prevent inadvertent contact, stay outside of arm's reach from each other during each entire drill.*

You will feel awkward practicing these at first. Practice them anyway: If you can't do these while privately practicing them with a training partner, you won't be able to on a dark street against a suspected Threat. You can also equip the role-playing "Threat" with a roll of coins held in a tight fist, as this is a useful weapon that is difficult to spot; if the defender can notice this, she should be able to notice a knife or a gun. Be able to see and observe a Threat's *fingers*. While alternating roles with your training partner and playing the Threat, try to be creative in how you conceal the "weapon" and what you can say or do to try to distract the role-playing Defender. Get to know your enemy. Remember if you are confronted with an actual weapon-bearing assailant, give up your valuables and flee as soon as possible.

The scenarios are intended to:

- Provide you with judgment by exposing you to common attack situations
- Get you accustomed to being aware of your surroundings (360 awareness)
- Help you get past your resistance to recognizing and responding to Threats

Find a location with a lot of space for you and your training partner to move around safely. Practice roll-playing these with **no physical contact** between participants. For all these, begin by practicing your scanning, awareness, and recognition skills.

1. Role-play with a "Threat" following you. Turn to face the Threat.

Practice verbal commands ("Back off!"), palms forward, fingers up. Threat complies. Once you are comfortable with this exercise, repeat the scenario with the stalker not complying until you toss simulated "valuables" off to his side. Then have the person role-playing the Threat try to conceal a non-hazardous, small object (representing a weapon) in one hand. **Watch hands.** Always be ready and eager to flee. **No physical contact.**

2. Defend your bubble. Set your protective radius' size at a distance from which you believe you can run away safely without the role-playing Threat catching you from behind. This radius depends on available space, your speed, the Threat's apparent abilities, and how far you have to run to get to safety. It is also a good idea to role-play a Threat attempting to approach within arm's reach (your Red Zone) while trying to distract the defender with conversation. Be rude. Be ready. Keep working your plan to escape: look all around for a potential accomplice. Defend your bubble by shouting and gesturing before the Threat can breach it. Move away when you can. Don't forget to check fingers for weapons. Use verbal commands, **Threat disengages**. **No physical contact** during this drill. RUDE IS THE NEW SAFE.

3. Try this scenario: you and the Threat get closer while walking in opposite directions. The threat makes momentary, friendly small talk to try to cause you to lower your alertness and appears to continue on his way. However, once you pass the Threat, he or she turns and approaches you from behind. Turn and use the verbal command and gestures you've just drilled. In some simulations, you can try equipping the attacker with a simulated weapon and practice that way. **No physical contact**.

4. Next, a "predator" is rushing up behind you with intent to tackle you to the ground. Using your awareness scanning skills, you sense and respond according to the situation: fleeing, verbal commands, shedding valuables. **No physical contact.**

5. Three-person drill: A robbery is also a common scenario. Role-play that you are approached from the front or side by a Threat accompanied by an accomplice approaching from behind. Use your peripheral vision

to notice then monitor both Threats. Keep moving to avoid getting trapped between them in order to make a path to flee. You comply (toss "valuables" somewhat past Threats to direct them away from you) and flee. Note: the way to fight multiple attackers is to *not* fight multiple attackers. Keep moving to try to keep one of them between you and the other so that only one at a time can be trying to attack you. To understand how dangerous multiple attackers can be, just stand between two cars with your training partners and imagine being approached from both directions at once with no escape path open. If you're unarmed, this is a situation that only the highest awareness and a great deal of training can save you from. **No physical contact.**

The Fight Is On: Adrenaline Flood

"When you're throwing techniques, it's your turn. When you stop throwing techniques, it's the other guy's turn. We don't like it when it's the other guy's turn." —undefeated middleweight full contact karate world champion Bill Wallace[89]

You want to stay one step ahead of a predator so you are able to surprise him—not the other way around as he's planned.

It is often said that adrenaline will prepare you for flight or fight, but people may choose neither of those options. Some will immediately surrender in an attempt to negotiate with or even befriend their attackers (a psychological phenomenon called Stockholm Syndrome). Yet another response can occur: During airliner cabin evacuations on the ground, despite flight attendants and pilots screaming, "Release your seat belts and get out!" as well as which exits to use, some passengers shut down in what's called "negative panic". They die in their seats, seat belts still fastened, looking straight ahead while the cabin fills with smoke. You don't know what you'll do until you're faced with

---

[89] Bill "Superfoot" Wallace workshop attended by the author at Karate College, Radford University, 1998. He was speaking of ring fighting.

a stressful situation, and this is why Athena Women presents attack scenarios so you can be more confident and better prepared to deal with stress.

Adrenaline:

- is your friend—for a few minutes
- makes more energy available to your major muscles
- reduces blood supply to the skin
- forces your rate of breathing to increase
- raises your heart rate

Combat stress (the belief you're about to be attacked)[90] can cause you to:

- not think clearly
- lose fine motor skills
- suffer tunnel vision
- not hear certain sounds

When you're tense, you:

- waste energy with subconsciously tightened muscles
- suffer from slower reactions
- telegraph your strikes
- tire quickly

---

[90] "Psychological Effects of Combat" (accessed January 13, 2016); available from http://www.ki llology.com/art_psych_combat.htm

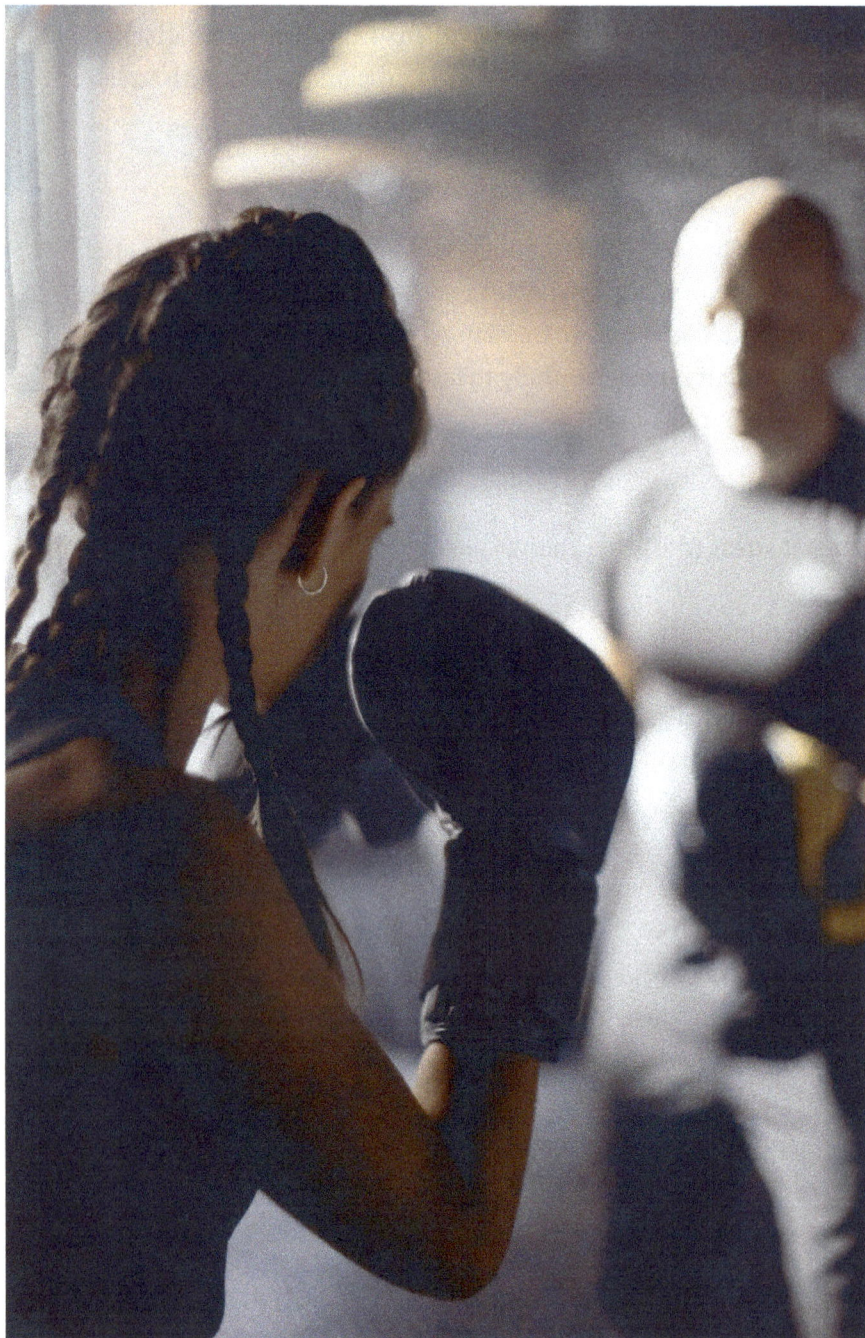

Training to fight back under duress. Photo: Cottonbro Studio

There is a lot going on here. In the above first group, adrenaline's effects prepare you to use your large muscles by taking in more oxygen and increasing your heart's pumping to distribute that extra oxygen. Lowering blood flow to your skin will conserve your blood quantity if you're injured and bleeding.

The second group of effects is why you should plan and train to use only simple fighting techniques. To be able to use any technique you must have practiced it enough times that it you can use it without your higher brain thinking about it. Often misnamed "muscle memory", you need to have done enough repetitions to have formed the *neural pathways* needed to execute a movement using only your lower-thinking brain. Techniques that require intricate movements will not be available to you during a violent confrontation—imagine trying to write neatly while terrified. Large muscle motor skills is all you'll be able to use. Tunnel vision and dampened hearing force you to focus on the Threat. For these reasons, you should only learn simple, gross-motor movements. Imagine trying to do arithmetic while being assaulted: We encourage you to practice each fighting technique you learn every other day *until it is as automatic as your startle reaction.* The number of reps necessary to reach that goal varies greatly by individual, but at minimum is several hundred repetitions and can require thousands. What's your life worth?

Stress can inflict the last group of the above on you. Tense muscles slow your reactions because the opposite muscles that should be relaxed while you're moving are tense and working against the movement you desire. Beginning a strike while you're tense is much more work as your body is working against itself so rather than using minimal energy for a strike—as Bruce Lee advocated—you waste energy. The result is awkward and slower movements that tell a predator you are beginning to move. Finally, being tense while fighting can exhaust you in mere seconds.

Recall what we said about taking initiative by having and executing a plan; it helps reduce anxiety and keeps your mind in the present and on your safety. Imagine for a moment that you are right now in a confrontation that is clearly about to turn violent. You're past any opportunities to flee, de-escalate or comply, you're trapped and will be physically assaulted within moments, and you have no other choice but to engage the assailant. ***Allowing a confirmed predator the opportunity to strike first is unacceptably dangerous***. Establishing and verbally defending your bubble, thereby positively identifying an encroaching Threat as now putting you in imminent danger of injury informs your next decisions.

Fight back ferociously enough (within the *reasonable force* rule) to compel an attacker to stop focusing on attacking you and start focusing on defending himself and worrying about the witness attention you're attracting. Force him to be unwilling to continue his assault.) It is more likely that you can make an attacker unwilling to continue his attack than you will make him unable to continue his attack by quickly injuring him enough. Don't let that discourage you: getting him to run away is a win. This is the difference between fighting to escape on the street versus fighting to win in a ring. In Liddy's way of thinking, **make your enemy worry about you.**

Post-Attack: Adrenaline Crash

What happens if the attacker is injured? A downed attacker might be playing possum, may recover quickly, or have friends nearby. If he ran away, he could return—with a weapon or accomplices. You'll have plenty of time to feel sorry for him (or not) later, in a safe place. Do not hang around to decompress there and then. Whether the attacker appears to be injured or has fled, **the final defensive step is to move away:** *flee toward safety.*

Complying With Police Instructions

If you happen to still be at the scene of an assault on you as the police arrive, recognize that the officers might not yet know what happened, *including whether you are a victim or a suspect who might be armed.* They need to assess, stop the situation from getting worse, decide whether to call for more officers or medical help, and secure the crime scene, all before starting their investigation into who did what. Slow down and let them do their jobs.

It is life-and-death crucial to follow the officers' instructions exactly

and immediately. Listen intentionally. In particular, if an officer tells you to "Keep your hands where I can see them," that would be *the worst time* to decide to reach into your pocket or purse for your phone. Following instructions will help the officers sort out what happened as quickly as possible. If you've injured someone—even if you've stayed within the law—do not be surprised if you get a free ride to the police station lockup.

Afterward

Answer questions about your experience only after you've recovered to a normal emotional state (according to a qualified observer, not yourself). Give yourself twenty-four hours or more. Make statements only in the presence of your attorney.

If you were involved in a physical altercation, get medical attention because your adrenaline may be masking injuries.

Our or other training, if taken post-attack *and conducted with the particular needs of a victim in mind*, helps restore confidence and a sense of control in victims but obviously an attack can remain traumatizing and call for different assistance in addition to what our training can provide. Check in with a counselor.

* * *

THIS [91] is a scripted training video of a woman role-playing an untrained person failing to assert herself, not fighting back, and ending up kidnapped. During the next run-through, she asserts herself by first challenging a male thug and then explosively fighting back using her extensive fighting training against the same attack by him and his male accomplice. Please take a few

---

[91] "Martial arts mom with baby VS. two kidnappers in Walmart parking lot..." (accessed November 10, 2023); available from https://www.youtube.com/watch?v=imfJtdlUaQY

minutes to view and ponder this video as follows:

View the first run of the scenario and write down anything you would have done differently as a result of what you've learned from this book. Only after you've done that, watch the second, corrected version of the attack and counterattack.

Kudos to you if you noticed that in all scenarios, while loading her vehicle, she stays focused on what she is doing to the exclusion of her environment. Obviously she needs to be careful with her "baby" but since she is trapped between the two vehicles she should also keep looking around. As a result of her task fixation, you see that the first "attacker" gets within grabbing distance of her before she is aware of him. However, this is a necessary part of the scenario to set up showing how she escapes from a double wrist grab.

Knowing what you've learned from this book, are there other actions you would take, beginning at the start of this scenario? Consider possible outcomes of those actions.

*Here's an example of a "what-if" situation one of our students experimented with. Walking along the sidewalk, daytime in a business district, she scanned and thanks to her new **awareness** skills noticed a group of males standing around some distance ahead of her. She chose to imagine that their behavior highlighted them as suspected Threats. She moved to the second step of our Five Step Plan, **avoidance**, and ducked into an open business. Immediately she realized that she had traded one problem for another. She was inside a business with other people nearby, a less likely site for harassment or an attack. However, she could no longer keep the group in sight, costing her some Situational Awareness, or SA. Had she not practiced that scenario, she would not have thought of this new problem. This led to the question of whether simply crossing the street would have been a safer option: **Learning occurred.** Also, now inside the store, if this was taking place during darkness with few passers-by, would she call someone or a taxi for a ride from the store to her car or would she step outside and proceed alone? What would you do?*

This is an example of the benefit of making self-protection a habit, which builds your confidence.

12

IS ONLINE SAFETY POSSIBLE?

"Privacy is the right to be left alone." —US Justice Louis Brandeis

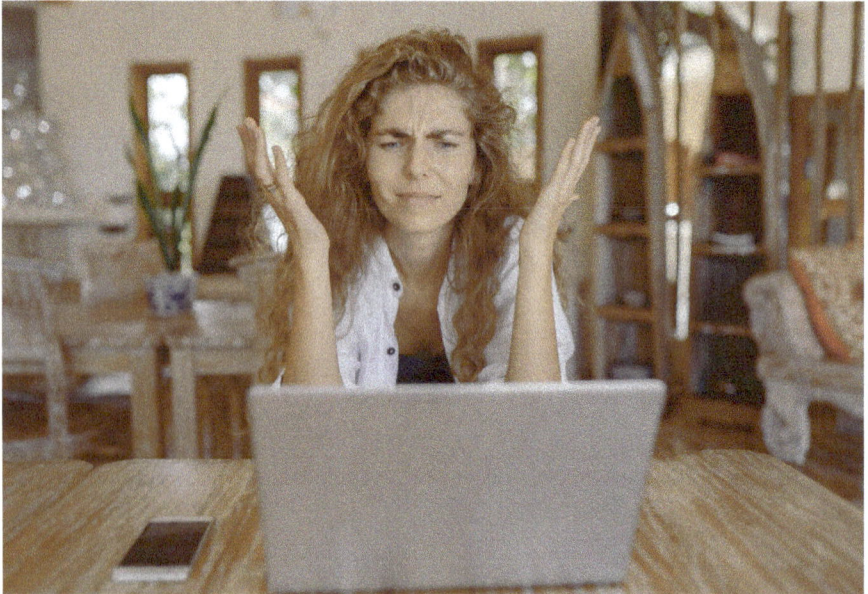

Photo: Yan Krukau

The excellent video, OBLIVIOUS, (https://www.youtube.com/watch?v=euc-WcN5IkY) *about online stalkers was produced by a young woman for her younger sister. In the comments, the big sister warns, "Not everyone is who they say they are." Forget Tinsel Town's products: this is worthy of Best Picture.*

Breaking news:
Watch THIS VIDEO BY ROB BRAXMAN, "The Internet Privacy Guy". (https://www.youtube.com/watch?v=nCFbgWjgp2M)

The biggest judgment error made by people when it comes to online data privacy is to assume that the data snoops only know what we've disclosed.

There is a sinister, growing use of online, scattered, personally identifiable information to try to threaten or ruin companies and individuals. Unless you've taken measures to be anonymous online (I show you how in this section), this means every social media post, everywhere you've traveled (political rally, medical specialist, etc.) while carrying your phone or paying electronically, every search term you've ever entered, your browsing history, your contacts list, emails you've sent or received and your entire YouTube account activity are stored. Yes, much of your personal data and habits has been saved without not only your consent, but sometimes without even your knowledge. What you do today is being added to what the digital spies and stalkers already know about you, perhaps to be used to attack or ostracize you—even years later. This is already occurring.

The motivation for vacuuming up and using our personal information is for the usual money and/or control. The crucial difference now is the use of online information to utterly destroy those who simply disagree with the data collectors. This shouldn't surprise us: try to name a technology that has not been weaponized or misused by someone—regardless of what political side you or they they are on. The guilty parties range from the lone hacker to some of the biggest corporations on the planet. Not to mention government mass data collection. As Lavrentiy Beria, Joseph Stalin's vicious head of secret police, said, "Show me the man and I will show you the crime."

Think about the non-PC jokes or memes or photos—even in jest—you've posted or simply given a thumbs-up on social media over the past decade or more. Comments about political candidates, groups that you've joined and items you've uploaded or reposted are all ripe for the picking. Each of your transgressions, no matter how trivial—because *nothing* is too trivial to these digitally empowered thugs—can be tabulated and assigned scores for: social, gender, energy, economic, green, religious, racial, political, climate or CO_2 "justice". You will be not just punished, but utterly banished from the public square *and economy.* Your legal-tender currency is already not usable on some payment platforms to do business with certain out-of-favor businesses or people.

This "canceling" or "shadow-banning" is already happening to companies. Self-appointed arbiters—whether local or national groups—are assigning companies scores in efforts to coerce them to change their business practices or stop doing business with those who are unapproved. Large companies— bullies—with near-monopolies on their services are refusing to do business with individuals or businesses with whom they simply disagree.

Likewise, this is already happening to individuals. We've seen news stories of people whose lives have been turned upside down because of a single online or public comment made years or decades earlier—regardless of the culture or context when and where the comment was made.

So you say you've done or said nothing that violates good character? According to whom, and by what standards in place at what time? ***You** do not get to decide what is unacceptable to the electronic mob.* They are prosecutor, judge, jury and executioner and you're shouted down when you attempt to defend your actions.

The Internet Never Forgets

As the late Dr. Kurt Richebäcker stated, there is a difference between data and information; he defined information as usable data. You may have said or done some particular thing in a certain situation during a different time with different norms, but if someone conceals these contextual factors, the digitized, sterilized record of that event is just meaningless data. Meaningless—but usable to be weaponized against you, so that you find it difficult to get a job you have worked toward, rent an apartment, get elected to your town council, open an account, or get admitted to your desired college if those operations lack the spine to stand up to the *petty little tyrants* that are being enabled by **mass data collection**. Data handling technology now enables both the compiling of your data and dissemination of tyrants' judgments of you. *Your reputation is now available and vulnerable world-wide.* You might be interested in gaining control of your personal information. Because it is *yours.* Not someone else's to beat you over your head with.

When faced with bulk collection of your personal information, rather than shrugging and retreating to "So what, I have nothing I need to hide from you," **put the onus back on the snoops where it belongs: "I've secured my information because *I have nothing I need to show you.*"** Since some of your personal information has already slipped its leash, why bother to control it now? As C. S. Lewis observed, "You can't go back and change the beginning, but but you can start where you are and change the ending."

* * *

"Trackers from different companies were communicating with each other to confirm the identity of visitors to a website for victims of sexual violence." [92]

Character counts: **Violating the privacy of victims who've already been severely violated by terrible crimes is an abomination**, and proof that the ethics of some slimy online data collectors have fled the scene. *If they stoop to*

---

[92] "The High Privacy Cost of a "Free" Website" (accessed October 30, 2020); available from https://themarkup.org/blacklight/2020/09/22/blacklight-tracking-advertisers-digital-priv acy-sensitive-websites

this, what won't they do to you? If ever there was an example of the need to become anonymous online, this is it.

* * *

"The scandal isn't how they're [governments and corporations that are collecting our data] breaking the law. The scandal is that they don't have to break the law."— *Edward Snowden on "The Joe Rogan Experience" podcast.*

"The right of the people to be secure in their persons, houses, papers, and effects, against unreasonable searches and seizures, shall not be violated, and no Warrants shall issue, but upon probable cause, supported by Oath or affirmation, and particularly describing the place to be searched, and the persons or things to be seized." —Fourth Amendment to the US Constitution.

* * *

"Website operators may agree to set cookies—small strings of text that identify you—from one outside company. But they are not always aware that the code setting those cookies can also load dozens of other trackers along with them, like nesting dolls, each collecting user data." [93] [Ahead I show you how to stop this easily.]

"Thanks to a new Vermont law requiring companies that buy and sell third-party personal data to register with the Secretary of State, we've been able to assemble a list of 121 data brokers operating in the U.S" [94]

---

[93] *Ibid.*

[94] "A landmark Vermont law nudges over 120 data brokers out of the shadows" (accessed April 26, 2021); available from https://www.fastcompany.com/90302036/over-120-data-brokers-inch-out-of-the-shadows-under-landmark-vermont-law

* * *

A business frequented by children was approached by an individual looking to place an ad on the company's website.

Fortunately the company's I.T. guru nosed around and discovered that the individual was a registered pedophile whose "ad" code was suspected to have been designed to hack into the company's computer system and steal data about the children enrolled there. Online anonymity is sounding better all the time.

* * *

Jaron Lanier (the "father of virtual reality") commented in the Netflix documentary movie *The Social Dilemma* that you are not the customer of social media, and that even categorizing your role as a product to sell to advertisers is too simplistic. Lanier believes that the result of social media is **"the gradual, slight, imperceptible change in your own behavior and perception"** (emphasis in the original). Some former social media designers interviewed said they do not allow their children to use social media. Are we amateurs smarter than these designers?

* * *

The Spread Privacy blog (operated by the privacy search engine and browser DuckDuckGo), makes a persuading argument for privacy by debunking the *I have nothing to hide* mentality. It reads in part, "...small pieces of personal data are increasingly aggregated by advertising platforms like Google and Facebook to form a more complete picture of who you are, what you do, where you go, and with whom you spend time. And those large data profiles can then lead much more easily to significant privacy harms. If that feels creepy, it's because it is." [95]

When tyrants come into power, they often take two actions: confiscate means of self-defense and trample on citizens' right to privacy by conducting searches. When you're online, people are trying to identify you and log everything you do (electronic searching and stalking)—to the point they can predict your actions and reactions. Imagine how much more of a threat this is when weaponizing AI.

Right now, much of the world wide web's default operating mode is **collecting your personal information, sometimes even to the degree of defeating measures you take to retain it**. This is the attitude of **criminal, human predators**: it is their duty to prey on you and it is yours to be defenseless prey. In my view, online predators play by the same rules: attack while conducting their schemes in the shadows, then work even harder to defeat you when you try to fight back. **Digital predators are waging a world war against privacy. And we are funding them.**

Privacy is a human need because it is in our private moments and spaces that we think and plan and communicate clearly and meaningfully.

Privacy is a human right and therefore must be the default operating premise of any system. Borrowing a popular phrase, *in human rights terms, the internet is an* epic fail.

* * *

"When you say, 'I don't care about the right to privacy because I have nothing

[95] "Three Reasons Why the 'Nothing to Hide' Argument is Flawed" (accessed November 2, 2020); available from https://spreadprivacy.com/three-reasons-why-the-nothing-to-hide-argument-is-flawed/

to hide,' that's no different than saying, 'I don't care about freedom of speech because I have nothing to say or freedom of press because I have nothing to write.'" —*Edward Snowden* [96]

* * *

How To Use This Section

Few things are more frustrating than asking a simple technology question and getting an answer that sounds like the machine language of ones and zeros—completely unintelligible to us humans. I've written this section for average people such as you and me who just want to take simple steps to reduce online risks.

At the end of this section are steps that you can take to be safer online, including tips on avoiding stalkers on social media.

What Threats Lurk Online?

Disclaimer: I am not trained in information technology or cyber security. The following discussion is a result of research I've done as well as the experience I have using precautions and privacy applications for various functions. If you choose to have better than the protection I advocate, consult a subject matter expert on IT security.

- *"29% of teens have been stalked or contacted by a stranger..."* [97]

---

[96] "Edward Snowden about Privacy" attributed to *The Guardian* (accessed January 12, 2020); available from https://www.youtube.com/watch?v=bpO3GeXTceM

[97] "30 Statistics about Teens and Social Networking" (accessed January 9, 2016); available from http://facebook-parental-controls-review.toptenreviews.com/30-statistics-about-teens-and-social-networking.html

- *"55% of teens have given out personal info to someone they don't know, including photos and physical descriptions."* [98]
- *According to the Family Online Safety Institute,15% of teens met someone in person with whom they had previous contact online.*

How do people or businesses use your online activities to discover personal information? What are you probably doing now that is making it easier for people to identify and track you—both online and physically? Do you know how to get control of your security and privacy?

Let's first talk about how easily corporations, governments and bad guys *identify* you and how they *track* your online activities to learn about you.

---

[98] "30 Statistics about Teens and Social Networking" (accessed January 9, 2016); available from http://facebook-parental-controls-review.toptenreviews.com/30-statistics-about-teens-and-social-networking.html

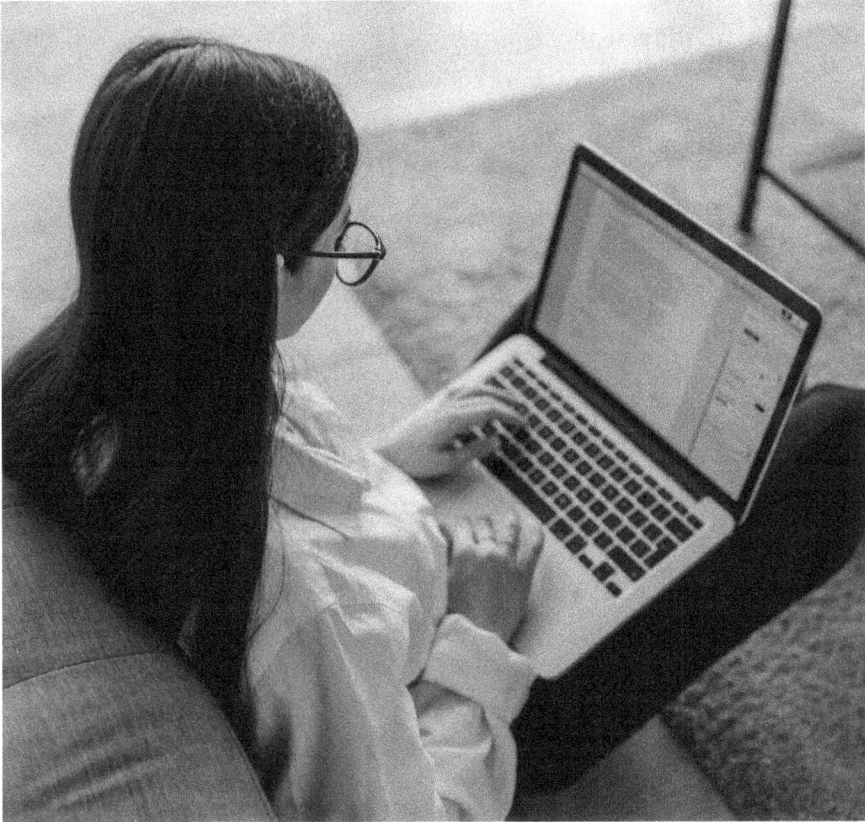

Photo: Vlada Karpovich

Who You Are: Want A Cookie?

Obviously a website you log into knows who you are. Cookies do different things, from simple to complex, according to the intent of the website host or owner. They identify you to the cookie's owner and can help you log in faster or save your settings. Third party cookies from sites you may have never visited are embedded in your device when the website you're visiting has agreed to do so for the other company in exchange for click-through revenue or exposure. A newer type of cookie, called LSOs (or Local Stored Objects) are being referred to as Super Cookies because of their capabilities and the fact they can last indefinitely, buried in your computer's files. In a disagreement, the side that controls the language of the debate often wins the argument. Naming software code that can allow websites to track you "cookies" was, in my view, a devious marketing masterstroke.

Who You Are: Internet Protocol & Device Identifiers

You visit the website of a company for the first and only time. You leave no personal information—or so you think. Just a few days later, advertising material from that company appears in your home's physical mailbox, personally addressed to you—also for the first time. You know this cannot be a coincidence. How did that company figure out who you are and where you live when all you did was visit their website for a few minutes?

The above incident happened to me. Later, I learned it was very easy for the company to find me. When you connect a device *directly* to the internet, it is assigned by your Internet Service Provider (ISP) an identifier that online devices use to find and communicate with each other. That identifier is called a public IP (Internet Protocol) address.[99] Anyone operating a website sees the public IP addresses of their visitors, and they can also track and find the physical location of an IP address (to see both your public IP address and your physical location, go to ip-tracker.org). You may have heard that every device that connects to the Internet has its own unique IP address, but that is not exactly the case. If you have a network in your home, your router is assigned the public IP address and your router then assigns a private IP address to each device on your home network. These private IP addresses are not reachable outside the range of your router.[100]

An even more specific identifier is embedded into smartphones, a number that, unlike an IP address, cannot be changed. "The use of these identifiers poses a greater risk than tracking technologies typically used on PC Web

---

[99] "What Is An IP Address?" (accessed January 4, 2016); available from http://computer.howstuffworks.com/internet/basics/question549.htm

[100] "How and Why All Devices in Your Home Share One IP Address" (accessed June 7, 2018); available from https://www.howtogeek.com/148664/how-and-why-all-devices-in-your-home-share-one-ip-address/

browsers, said Heng Xu, an assistant professor of information sciences and technology at Pennsylvania State University. This is because the numbers are difficult or impossible to delete and can be tied to other data, like a person's location at a given moment, she said. Matching the phone identifier to these other types of information 'poses a serious threat to consumer privacy,' Ms. Xu said." [101]

So far, corporations know your public IP address but they may not yet know who you are. Then you visit a website that offers you a discount coupon for signing up with your email address (sound familiar?). Or you open a store account to buy things online. You get a discount for revealing your email address, and now all your data that has already been associated with that email address is connected to your public IP address. *Gotcha.* (The company that mailed me advertising saw my IP and connected that with my online profile that other companies have built on me.) "Today, email is identity. Your email address is the one common thread that ties together all the various services you use online and serves as your username or unique identifier stating who you are across the entire internet."[102] ProtonMail [103] and DuckDuckGo [104] offer ways to email with parties that you don't trust to protect your privacy without providing them with your actual email address.

How Websites Follow You

"The websites that track you use three main methods: **cookies, fingerprint-**

---

[101] "Unique Phone ID Numbers Explained" (accessed March 22, 2016); available from http://blogs.wsj.com/digits/2010/12/19/unique-phone-id-numbers-explained/

[102] Yen, Andy, "Email is more than communication – It's your identity and worth protecting," (accessed September 27, 2023); available from https://proton.me/blog/email-is-your-digital-id

[103] "Secure Mail That Protects Your Privacy" (accessed November 10, 2023); available from https://proton.me/mail

[104] "DuckDuckGo Email Protection" (accessed November 10, 2023); available from https://duckduckgo.com/duckduckgo-help-pages/email-protection/duck-addresses/

ing, and **beacons**." [105]

Where You Go Online: Tracking Cookies

If you take your phone, tablet, or laptop to a different WiFi network your phone's public IP address will change. Corporations can still track you. If you take your phone or laptop to another network, the cookies that have been planted on your device still tell their Websites who you are. How many cookies might be on your device? The browser without extra privacy protections in the desktop computer I'm using to write this had a few minutes ago 852 cookies planted in it by websites—some of which I've never visited.

Where You Go Online: Fingerprinting

Websites may also discern who you are by looking at the combination of settings you use in your browser. You make the effort to retain anonymity and privacy online by carefully configuring your software. Then slimy data collectors come up with a way to try to *violate your privacy* by specifically trying to defeat the steps you take to protect yourself. Had enough yet?

Where You Go Online: Trackers

There are trackers that operate from web pages. Web beacons—tiny files embedded in web pages—report what you click on back to the website so they learn your interests. "Conversion tracking—measuring how many people actually go on to buy or do something with a site after clicking through an advert—is a method long used by the likes of Google and Microsoft to grease their ad engines and ultimately generate more cash from marketing

---

[105] What is Internet Tracking? (and How To Avoid Being Tracked) (accessed October 31, 2020); available from https://choosetoencrypt.com/search-encrypt/internet-tracking-why-its-bad-and-how-to-avoid-it/

campaigns." [106] "Google is still collecting information to serve us ads. In fact, we recently told you how Google is tracking the websites you visit and the videos you watch to better understand your interests." [107]

Beware Your Email Inbox

"Tracking pixels [*also known as web beacons—SL*] and cookies aren't the only way companies spy on you. Tracking links in emails tell the sender what emails you opened and what you clicked. They use this information to personally identify you, profile your interests, and follow your behavior across apps and websites.

"With our new Tracking Links Protection feature, we now detect and clean known tracking links, directing you safely to the web page without surveillance. Proton Mail is the first email service to offer this level of protection because we believe your inbox belongs to you." [108]

"The Creepy Line"

Popular search engines[109] record the searches done by you and save them to a profile that corporations build on you.[110]

If you were shopping in your local mall, would you allow every store you visit to assign someone to follow you and attach sticky notes to your coat, spelling out your name, your home and email address, your shopping habits

[106] "Facebook: 'We didn't patent stalking logged-off users'" (accessed January 5, 2016); available from http://www.theregister.co.uk/2011/10/04/facebook_patent_conversion_tracking/

[107] "3 search sites that don't track you like Google does" (accessed January 5, 2016); available from http://www.komando.com/tips/251012/3-search-sites-that-dont-track-you-like-google-does/all

[108] Email from Proton, August 18, 2023.

[109] "5 Alternative Search Engines That Respect Your Privacy" (accessed October 31, 2020); available from https://www.howtogeek.com/113513/5-alternative-search-engines-that-respect-your-privacy/

[110] "Don't Track Us" (accessed January 4, 2016); available from http://donttrack.us.

and preferences, what you bought, and even what you only looked at? Not only that, but these notes would be displayed for everyone to see. The notes stay attached to you after you leave the mall, and everywhere you go more notes mysteriously get stuck on you—even after visiting a physician or counselor or attorney. Each subsequent place you visit would immediately have your personal information and add more notes to your coat. By the time you finish your day, you'd be covered in sticky notes and everyone you meet would know what was written on them. Would you permit such creepy, stalking behavior? Well, **this is the real-world equivalent to what's happening to you while you are online.**

Some "free" online services—such as Gmail (Google)—automatically scan your emails then show you advertisements relating to what's in those messages. Using your information to target you with ads is how Google makes money from their "free" services. Facebook doesn't sell your information to marketers; instead it sells to the marketers *access* to you without revealing your identity.[111]

According to the DuckDuckGo's Spread Privacy blog, their "data set shows Google-owned trackers are on over 85% of the top 50K sites and Facebook on 36%…" Furthermore, DuckDuckGo's research finds that only approximately one out of five people use tracker protection of any quality. Their privacy mobile browsers and browser extensions include tracker blocking.[112]

"We don't need you to type at all. We know where you are. We know where you've been. We can more or less know what you're thinking about," said Google's former CEO Eric Schmidt. He also stated (irony alert), "Google policy is to get right up to the creepy line and not cross it." [113]

Facebook has a history of intruding into your privacy and has had to reverse

---

[111] "What You Can Do About Facebook Tracking" (accessed January 5, 2016); available from http://www.wsj.com/articles/what-you-can-do-about-facebook-tracking-1407263246.

[112] "DuckDuckGo Tracker Radar Exposes Hidden Tracking" (accessed November 5, 2020); available from https://spreadprivacy.com/duckduckgo-tracker-radar/

[113] "Google's CEO: 'The Laws Are Written by Lobbyists'" (accessed January 5, 2016); available from http://www.theatlantic.com/technology/archive/2010/10/googles-ceo-the-laws-are-written-by-lobbyists/63908/

some of those invasions; Canadian and German government officials have accused the platform of violating their laws.[114]

"Facebook is following you," says *The Wall Street Journal*.[115] More: "Facebook rolled out its new policies and terms on January 30th, 2015. In the text, Facebook authorizes itself to (1) track its users across websites and devices; (2) use profile pictures for both commercial and non-commercial purposes and (3) collect information about its users' whereabouts on a continuous basis. Facebook announced the changes more than a month in advance, but the choice for its one billion and rising users remained the same: agree or leave Facebook." [116]

Would you let someone you don't know look over your shoulder while you are online or physically follow (i.e.,stalk) you *everywhere* you go? As of 2015, Facebook tracked you after you visited any page on their domain—even if you were not a member, and sometimes you didn't even have to visit a Facebook page.[117]

We have to decide and work to hang on to our privacy. Fortunately people, companies and some officials in Europe and California are finally starting to push back on intrusions. Your personal information is just that: *personal* and *yours*.

One way to limit some of the tracking Websites do is to clean up your cookies, and there are browser settings and apps that limit or delete them for you.

Whatever you post on social media is *permanent* and *public*. Even with security settings protections, people can email, screenshot, or photograph

---

[114] "Protect Yourself Online," *Consumer Reports*, June, 2011, 26.

[115] "What You Can Do About Facebook Tracking" (accessed January 9, 2016); available from http://www.wsj.com/articles/what-you-can-do-about-facebook-tracking-1407263246

[116] KU Leuven Centre for IT & IP Law and iMinds-SMIT advise Belgian Privacy Commission in Facebook investigation (accessed January 7, 2016); available from http://www.law.kule uven.be/citip/en/news/item/icri-cir-advises-belgian-privacy-commission-in-facebook-investigation

[117] "Facebook 'tracks all visitors, breaching EU law'" (accessed January 9, 2016); available from http://www.theguardian.com/technology/2015/mar/31/facebook-tracks-all-visitors-breaching-eu-law-report

your posts and then re-post them for the world to see. It is an electronic form of gossiping, but more accurate. Remember, too, that potential employers look at your social media.

Hacking And Stalking

A few years ago, I saw news reports that photos of a scantily-clad young woman had scandalously found their way all over the internet—onto thousands of sites. At that time she was only fourteen years old. Any adults who were lustfully viewing the images of this juvenile were therefore effectively pedophiles. Are you creeped out yet? Don't post anything in a presumably private account that you wouldn't want to see on a highway billboard in your town.

Right now might be a fine time to prune your social media posts.

Radio, television and print ads are placed and paid for by advertisers who know that some of the people exposed to their ad will not be interested. That wastes money. With web tracking, advertisers can individually target their ads to you based on your known interests.

Who cares if companies know my personal information and track where I am?

"...the general manager of Uber New York Josh Mohrer told a journalist that [the individual] was both tracking her Uber ride and had accessed her ride-history logs without her permission." [118] *In this case, an employee used company data improperly and was able to track (stalk?) a customer. Also, "[i]n 2014, Uber discovered that a security breach had exposed the data of 50,000 drivers across the US."* [119] Uber later began encrypting customer data—after the data breach.

More recently regarding Uber: "[t]he company came clean on Tuesday

---

[118] "'God View': Uber Investigates Its Top New York Executive For Privacy Violations" (accessed April 27, 2021); available from https://www.buzzfeednews.com/article/johanabhuiyan/uber-is-investigating-its-top-new-york-executive-for-privacy#.vbJB3YKj4

[119] "Uber fined $20K in data breach, 'god view' probe" (accessed January 7, 2016); http://www.cnet.com/news/uber-fined-20k-in-surveillance-data-breach-probe/

[November 21, 2017] about its cover-up of a year-old hacking attack that stole personal information of about 57 million customers and drivers." [120] And, "…there are already pressing questions that demand swift answers. Who exactly within Uber's staff knew about the hack after it occurred, and how many people were actively involved in the cover-up, which involved paying the hackers $100,000 to delete data and keep the breach quiet?" [121]

* * *

Is This The World We Want To Create And Live In?

---

[120] "The Latest: States investigate Uber over massive data breach" (accessed January 11, 2018); available from https://www.washingtontimes.com/news/2017/nov/22/the-latest-uk-says-any-uber-fine-would-be-higher-t/

[121] "Uber Paid Off Hackers to Hide Massive Data Breach" (accessed January 11, 2018); available from https://www.technologyreview.com/s/609539/uber-paid-off-hackers-to-hide-massive-data-breach/

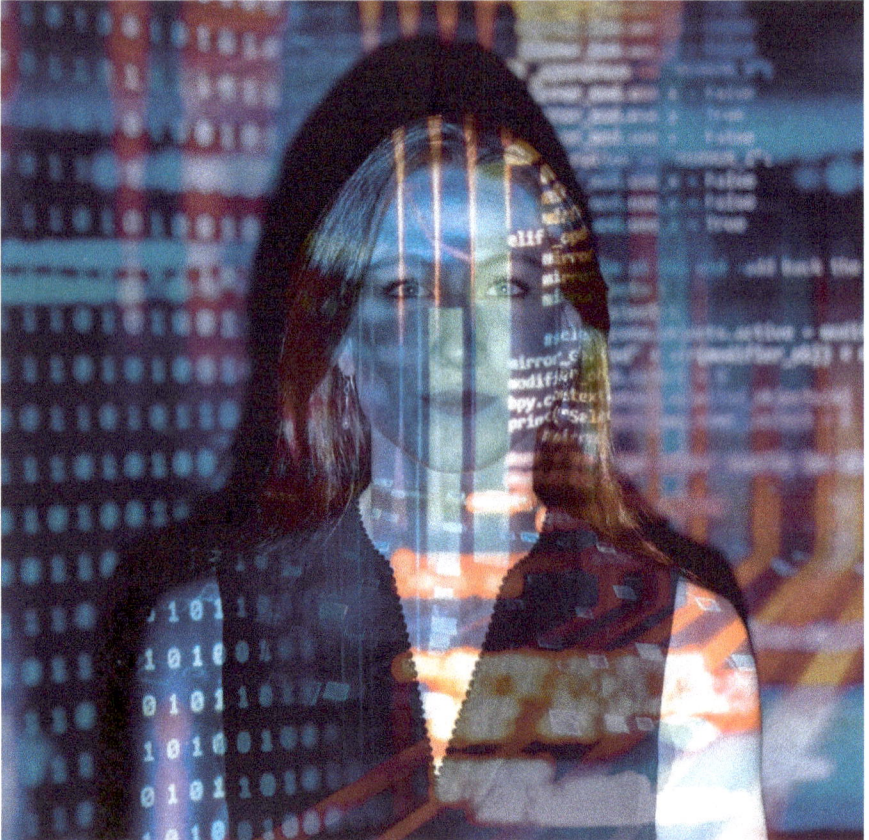

Photo: ThisIsEngineering

To dehumanize is to take away from a person what makes her or him human or individual. Privacy is a human quality and need, so depriving you of privacy is a step in depriving you of your humanity. Where do we end up if we continue walking this path?

There are three points here:

First, it's easy for companies—not to mention governments—to gather a lot of information about you. Second, your information is also useful to people and organizations with evil intent and sometimes they get hold of your information by improperly using or hacking into those many company or government databases in which you unwittingly appear. Third, whatever you post on social media can be useful to stalkers.

We don't have to be criminals to not want the world to know what medications we are taking, who our closest friends are and what we talk about with them, who we are dating, what our likes and dislikes are, what political party we favor, which physicians we see, where we are minute-by-minute or where we frequently travel. We close our curtains when we change our clothes, and we don't want strangers to hear our private phone calls or read our emails. Some people claim they're not worried about privacy—nonsense: they do not post the password for their email account online, do they?

How They Know Your Location

There are yet other ways you can be tracked. It's not just what sites you look at online, but where you physically go when you have your connected device with you. Remember: physical location of your device is easy to detect using your IP address (masking your device's IP address with a VPN may not hide your physical location from all *apps*, as some may use WiFi and/or GPS).[122] Your location might be harder for trackers to figure out if you use your browser instead of apps. Yes, security costs some inconvenience.

You may also be aware that almost all smartphone cameras record file data in every photograph's image. This contains information such as when the photo was taken, the camera's settings, and the GPS coordinates (location). That location data is sometimes referred to as a geotag. Normally, you can disable the geotag function so the location where photographs are taken is not stored in the picture's file.

If you don't disable the geotags and you upload to Facebook, the location data is uploaded, too. Anyone who can see your photo on that site can download it to get its location data. "...[O]ften apps like Facebook, Instagram, Twitter, and other photo sharing and social network applications will attempt

---

[122] "What Facebook Knows about you ... Part 1/2" (accessed January 9, 2016); available from http://blog.cubeyou.com/what-facebook-knows-about-you

to embed GPS data as well. If you don't want that to happen, pay more attention to what apps you allow to access your location data, and disable the ones you don't want to embed geographic coordinates with. You can use apps to remove all GEO and EXIF data as well, even after that data has been embedded into a picture." [123] Consider not allowing camera and social media apps to access your phone's location.

What About People With Evil Intent?

On New Year's Day 2016, police arrested and charged a man with stalking and weapons offenses. At the time police arrested him he was going to meet a girl he'd met on Facebook.[124] Good save by the police.

Geotagging photographs gives predators ways to find you. First, if you post a photo as soon as you take it, on a beach vacation for instance, you've revealed where you are in real time. Second, if you frequently upload photos during your normal activities, then a person stalking you will learn your routine and know when to expect you to be in various locations—not to mention he will know where you live if you take photos at home. The convenience of this location tagging is that you'll always know where you were when you took your pictures. If you do want your location data captured in your vacation photos, then why not wait until you're back home to upload them to social media? While you're taking pictures around your home and town where you don't need that data, disable your camera's geotag function. Remember, with or without photographs or geotags, if you update your "status" or "check in" online with your location, *you are helping predators find you.* If you mention that you're on a family outing, then you're telling everyone that your house is empty and ripe for burgling. Keep your family privately informed of your

---

[123] "How to See the Exact Location Where a Photo was Taken with a Mac" (accessed January 6, 2016); available from http://osxdaily.com/2015/05/08/view-exact-location-photo-taken-preview-mac/

[124] "Police: Armed Indiana Man Was Stalking Facebook 'Girlfriend' " (accessed January 1, 2016); available from http://abc13.com/news/indiana-man-arrested-for-stalking-facebook-girlfriend/1143142/

whereabouts; your hundreds of "friends" on social media can wait a few days.

Obsession: "Everyone Is Not Just Like Me"

Obsession: a persistent, disturbing preoccupation with an often-unreasonable idea or feeling.[125]

Most stalkers know their victims. Most stalkers are also young-to-middle age and already have a history of failed relationships. "Virtually anyone can be a stalker, just as anyone can be a stalking victim." [126] There are several types of stalkers; some more likely to attack, or rape you or even harm your loved ones to hurt you indirectly.[127,128] A stalker may be just someone awkward who doesn't know better, or they can be a dangerous stranger, acquaintance, or someone you had a relationship with. Stalkers can be serial stalkers, predator stalkers or love-obsessed stalkers, to name a few. A defining characteristic is persistence even after you've declined advances.

According to Laura Richards, CEO of the UK's Paladin National Stalking Advocacy Service, "Our cases range from victims being stalked from anything from six months to a staggering 22 years. Research shows that victims typically endure 100 incidents before they even call the police...Stalking is about fixation and obsession." [129]

Stalkers can be killers, and you can't diagnose which type is pursuing you. While a stalker might start following you after seeing you in person, he could also

---

[125] Webster's *Ninth New Collegiate Dictionary*, Springfield: Merriam Webster, Inc. 1985

[126] "Who Are Stalkers?" (accessed February 8, 2016); available from https://safeconnections.or g/who-are-stalkers/

[127] "Mind of a Stalker: Why Torment Someone?" (accessed February 7, 2016); available from http://www.webmd.com/sex-relationships/features/mind-stalker-why-torment-someon e

[128] "Forms of Stalking" (accessed February 7, 2016); available from http://www.esia.net/Forms_ of_Stalking.htm

[129] Laura Richards, "Rejected, obsessed and erotomanic: Inside the mind of a stalker" (accessed February 8, 2016); available from http://www.telegraph.co.uk/women/womens-life/1157717 6/Stalking-Rejected-obsessed-and-mentally-ill.-How-stalkers-think.html

become obsessed by just seeing you online (remember that Facebook says it can use your profile photo for its business activities, so some change their profile photo to a picture of their pet or some object). Seeing you—in person or online—can trigger someone with a stalker's mindset into obsession. You can't hide under a rock to keep weirdos from seeing you in person but together with the cooperation of your family and friends, *you can control* your online exposure. ***A stalker cannot obsess over you if he does not know you exist.***

If your online accounts have been compromised (hacked) or if you suspect you're being watched, stalked, or cyber-bullied—if someone is paying more attention to you than you're comfortable with—immediately let your family know. Law enforcement, counseling, and technical assistance may be needed, so do not hesitate to seek help.

Being stalked can be dangerous and also can affect mental health.[130] Don't be one of those victims who waits until she's been harassed or frightened hundreds of times before enlisting professional intervention.

$$* * *$$

Checklists: Improving Your Online Safety

This section does not consider the additional precautions you need to take if you're carrying your phone, tablet, computer or other device to a country where security, privacy or safety concerns exist (for a brief discussion of this, see the following chapter, The World Traveler).

Here is a **simple** site that will answer in plain language your questions about

---

[130] "Impact of stalking on victims" (accessed February 8, 2016); available from https://www.sta lkingriskprofile.com/victim-support/impact-of-stalking-on-victims

staying safe online: https://www.staysafeonline.org/stay-safe-online/. My quick tips follow.

To avoid getting bogged down, take these steps one at a time:

- Obviously the below cautions about providing your email address and phone number do not include businesses you trust, such as your medical caregivers.

- **Two important cyber security principles**: marketers and crooks cannot sell or lose control of your personal data if they do not have it. And you alone decide to whom you provide *your* personal data. It belongs only to you.

- **Stop giving away your email address or phone number** to people or companies you have no relationship with in exchange for "free" junk you'll never use or to vote in a meaningless "survey" no one cares about. The purpose of such distractions: to get your personal information. I no longer deal with online outfits that do not need but still demand my email address or phone number in order to do business with them. Alternatives are is to have a spam-only, throw-away free email address that you never open and use (xxx)-555-1212 as your phone number.

- Especially if you're an Android user, **minimize the number of apps you download** and instead use your browser to connect to services. Apps— especially free ones— can drain battery power by repeatedly connecting your device to the internet. These connections are how apps send your personal information to their creators, who sell it. For any that you want to install, read their privacy policies and see how many needlessly *access the internet and your personal information* such as bookmarks, contacts list, calendar, location and so on. Is the app's function worth a deluge of spam and robocalls? When you no longer need an app, delete it. Note: apps that access the internet and your contact list may submit your friends and family members to a tsunami of new marketing harassment.

· Have **current hardware with the latest security protections**, such as your home's modem and router. An older router may not be as secure as a newer unit. Also be sure to check reviews online. You can get apps that watch for malware. I use Malwarebytes.

· **Keep your software updated**, including security software. You can read the latest reviews of security software for PCs and Macs online at *Consumer Reports, Cnet* and elsewhere.

· **Suggested settings for your browsers** (these settings may be found within your browser's menu, or in your system's/smartphone's Settings app): block third-party cookies, sometimes referred to as "prevent cross-site tracking", use https where available. In iOS Safari, turn off Safari Suggestions. Limit your devices' location-sharing per your preferences. In Apple devices, you can set location-sharing on, off, only allow when the app is in use, or ask your permission for each site or app that wants to use your location. All browsers have pluses and minuses.

- **You might want to consider switching from Google's Chrome to privacy browsers (such as Brave or DuckDuckGo) or install free privacy and security add-ons for your non-Google browser** that erase cookies when you close your browser and those that block ads and trackers (content blockers).

Content blockers block ads and trackers, but not cookies—these are handled separately by your browser's settings. These blocker add-ons are often referred to as browser extensions; check your browser's menu bar or your system's setting menu under Privacy. There are plenty of these available for Safari, Firefox and TOR (The Onion Router) browsers. For **Safari**, content blocker apps such as **Wipr** are a fine option.

If you want to police your cookies yourself, go to either your browser's menu or your device's Settings app, find a choice dealing with cookies, privacy or labeled Advanced. you should be able to view a list of data that websites have smuggled into your device—delete these at will. Obviously, this isn't a one-and-done task; any time you're online you will attract cookies unless you use a "block all cookies" setting, or **use a privacy window or setting that erases cookies upon closing the window or the browser**.

Note: deleting all cookies (manually or by installing an extension or browser that erases cookies when you close your browser or setting your browser to block all cookies) will probably mean you'll have to manually log in to some sites each visit. Once you remove a site's cookies, it can't recognize you as a return customer. Blocking all cookies may also make it impossible to stay logged into some sites if the web host uses what are called "session cookies". For more convenience, only delete those you don't recognize or don't want following you around, and visit trusted sites using a non-private window in your browser. You will almost certainly see Facebook and several Google items installed in your device—even if you never visit any of these places. Safari and the **Brave** browser offer normal and "privacy" windows. The latter erase all cookies when they close. **Keeping it simple**: I use the normal windows, that allow cookies to persist, for trusted sites such as my encrypted email service so that I don't have to login for each visit. Privacy windows are for all other sites so those cookies are erased upon closing those windows.

- **Use search engines that respect your privacy, such as**: family-friendly Swisscows https://swisscows.com/en or https://duckduckgo.com or https://www.qwant.com/ or https://www.mojeek.com/ (Mojeek is a UK based search engine and will return mostly non-US sites) or the Brave browser's native search engine. Most browsers will let you set one or more of them as the default search engine, or bookmark them for convenient use. They work like the search engines you're used to, except they don't track you or add to your online profile. As mentioned earlier, DuckDuckGo's privacy browsers and extensions include tracker blocking.

- **Install a Virtual Private Network (VPN) app**. Complicated name, but easy to use. Use of these is growing because now they're now simple to download and install.

VPNs mainly do two things: they **encrypt *all* your data stream** starting right at your device and **one of their servers steps in and takes your place (substitutes for your real IP address) to preserve your anonymity**. The results are that the hacker intercepting your encrypted WiFi data stream at the coffee house or hotel can't read it—your encrypted data stream "tunnel" appears as gibberish. Anyone attempting to use your IP address to either identify you and record your browsing interests or learn your physical location cannot. A VPN securely encrypts *all communications* into and out of your device by all apps, not just your browsers. Some VPNs also block malware, ads, and/or trackers.

Note: VPNs cannot save you from your apps, if you have installed apps that vacuum up your personal data, contact list, calendar, search engine and browser history, and physical location and upload it all to the app companies to sell. Access social media with a browser equipped with a content blocker, use a VPN, and adjust your settings to restrict what apps you allow to access your location. Look for a VPN that doesn't keep logs of your activity and has been around for a while and gets good reviews. As with everything else on the internet, I am leery of "free" software because that usually means you pay with your privacy. I like **https://protonvpn.com/**, which offers both free and paid service.

· Do *not* connect to a public WiFi unless you are using either a VPN or the **TOR Network browser** (https://www.torproject.org/). Think of TOR as a VPN that works only with the TOR browser. The free TOR browser says it "...allows you to improve your privacy and security on the Internet."[131] The TOR browser only encrypts your data and hides your communications to preserve anonymity (changes your IP address) when using the TOR browser itself. Other connections—such as other apps or other browsers—remain vulnerable unless you're also using a VPN. In addition to that, since the TOR network is a bunch of servers scattered around the world and relays your data through at least three of them, you'll notice some loss of speed. VPNs may slow you down a tiny bit, but in my experience less than the TOR browser does. The main attraction of TOR is that it is free.

· Use **strong passwords**, and different passwords for your accounts.

· Use **two- or three-factor identification** with accounts that offer this

---

[131] "About TOR Browser" (accessed January 12, 2020); available from https://tb-manual.torproj ect.org/about/

feature.

- On many devices with GPS installed, you can set up your phone so that it can be found from a computer by your **family members** who know your account info. (http://www.ehow.com/how_5335830_track-phone-show-exact-location.html) This is one way to let your family know where you are as long as your phone is with you.

- Photos taken with devices equipped with GPS often put location data in the picture's image file. Anyone who has a copy of that photo file, sometimes even if they downloaded it, can see when and where it was taken unless you **disable the location function of the camera or refuse permission for the camera *and social apps* to use your location**.

- You can check to see if your connection to a given website is secure: Look for either a little *closed* padlock icon in the URL address bar, the word "private", or the URL address begins with http**s** instead of http. That "s" means the connection is secure (encrypted). On some browsers you need to click on the address bar to see the *https* part of the URL.

- **Secure, encrypted offshore cloud storage is available**. What you're looking for is encryption that begins at your device, not at their server, where it could be compromised. And preferably hosted in a country with strong privacy laws, and not located in the "Five Eyes"[132] nations (US, Canada, Australia, New Zealand, UK). Suggestions: https://tresorit.com/individuals. Proton now also offers a secure, private cloud service.

- If you need to send a secure, encrypted email or attachment to anyone or just want **better email privacy**, SendInc is an easy and free way to do that, using your existing email service. https://www.sendinc.com. There are also many encrypted stand-alone email services and, again, you might want to choose one not based in any of the "Five Eyes" countries. Unfortunately SendInc is based in the US. Here is a list of privacy-focused email services.

Are you curious about the trackers, third party cookies, keystroke loggers or other types of tracking technologies hidden on specific web pages you visit? Just visit this site and type in the website you're curious about and hit Enter.

Also, the Brave browser and the DuckDuckGo browser and extension will display what trackers they are blocking on each website you visit.

Here Are Some Hints If You Decide To Continue Using Social Media:

- I avoid Google, Facebook (and Instagram and WhatsApp) for a number of reasons.

- CAUTION: Your privacy settings can be partially negated if any of your

---

dozens or hundreds of "friends" share your posts and photos on their pages, or take screenshots of your posts and personal information and repost, text, or email them.

- Replace Facebook with privacy respecting MeWe. If Facebook's and Google's information policies bother you, try Gab for genuine free speech. Gab also offers GabPay that replaces the payment outfits that censor us.

- To check and set your Facebook[133] privacy settings, click the padlock in the upper right of the screen and go through the pages on the menu, including the "See More Settings" and "Privacy Settings" links.

- Rather than your full name, consider using use only your first and middle names—or a nickname—as some users do or change the spelling of your last name.

- On a social site's profile page, do *not* enter your address or date of birth.

- Do *not* discuss where you live, which school you attend or where you work. Don't help stalkers find you.

---

[133] https://www.facebook.com/about/basics/what-others-see-about-you/

· If you belong to sites that have usernames, pick a different one for each site so predators can't as easily put together information on you.

· If a site won't let you register without giving your birthday, consider changing something in the date so identity thieves won't have that important piece of information.

· Do not post your plans or schedules on social sites. Public schools post their athletic schedules online so discussing your school name and sport can tell a dangerous person where you will be.

· Do not friend, message, text, tweet, chat, email, arrange dates, exchange photos or personal information or talk on your phone with anyone on your personal social media accounts you're not *positive* you *personally* know. Sex offenders set up social media pages with fake names and stolen profile pictures. Avoid the social media sites that make this stalking easier. If you must use social media for a business, open a separate account for that, posting only your minimum necessary, professional information and use it only for business.

Recovering Your Cyber Safety

The above suggestions are intended to make it more difficult for bad actors to violate your cyber privacy and security. If you are already a victim of those crimes (particularly after you've tried to secure your online presence) more aggressive actions may be needed. Your problem could be two-pronged:

apprehending or at least stopping the *person* committing the stalking, hacking or cyber bullying, and closing whatever *technical gaps* the miscreant found or created. Always report crimes including harassment and cyber stalking to law enforcement. This may be your first experience with a cyber criminal, but they know how to deal with such reprobates.

From "DuckDuckGo Privacy Weekly for August 24, 2023":

"Researchers at Adalytics found that one of Google's ad-targeting systems ran a banking ad on a popular YouTube children's show. 'As a result, leading tech companies could have tracked children across the internet, raising concerns about whether they were undercutting a federal privacy law'", the New York Times stated.

https://www.nytimes.com/2023/08/17/technology/youtube-google-children-privacy.html

And...

"A POLITICO analysis of every [U.S.] state privacy law passed in 2023 shows that the tech industry has notched a steady series of wins. In Oregon and the six other states that passed legislation between January and July, lawmakers enacted bills that bore clear hallmarks of lobbying influence."

https://www.politico.com/news/2023/08/16/tech-lobbyists-state-privacy-laws-00111363

* * *

The woman in THIS VIDEO[134] was terrorized for six months by an online stalker who found her through her social media pages. He made several threats to come to her workplace and eventually began threatening to rape her. She reports sleeping with a knife under her pillow and that she walked outdoors with her hand on her cellphone (which is not a security device). Note her extensive use of social media and that she'd hooked together all her social

---

[134] "The Inside Story: Woman terrorized by an online stalker"(accessed Novembef 10, 2023); available from https://www.youtube.com/watch?v=1jYk9JWwgl4

media accounts, simplifying the stalker's job of tracking her.

Each week, take one step from the checklists in this chapter to begin claiming your online privacy.

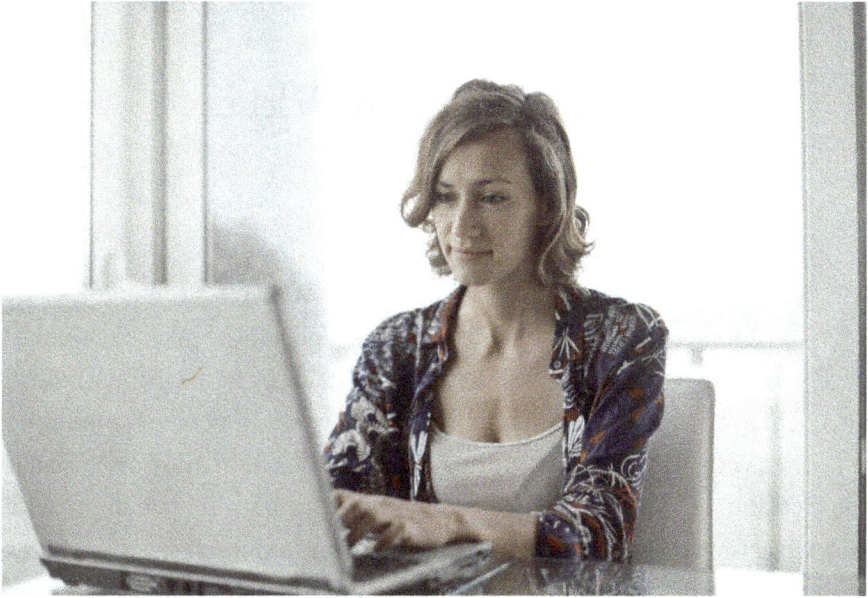

Photo: Andrea Piacquadio

13

THE WORLD TRAVELER

W hen traveling, especially through or to questionable locales, there are additional precautions you should take. Remember that you are a guest. Respect and abide by local customs, which also helps you avoid drawing attention to yourself. If you're traveling to countries with different dress norms, why not pack light and buy abroad if the clothing and US customs fees are within your budget? When my wife and I vacationed in Europe, we intentionally stayed in places the natives took their "holidays"; we rented vacation apartments away from tourist destinations. We rarely saw other Americans or heard English. After not seeing other Americans for a while, they stand out—and that can make you a target of criminals.

It is especially important to assimilate if you plan to visit poorer areas; do not wear jewelry or carry an expensive phone or camera in the open. Stay together. Plan ahead and know directions and train and bus schedules to facilitate return before nightfall if called for. Know where you're going, walk purposefully, and try not to need to ask directions. Check on the self-defense laws in the countries you will visit. Ask your hotel concierge for advice about where and when to walk around and what areas or times to avoid. Some criminals target tourists (who are unlikely to return to give testimony in court) for robberies and sexual assaults so stay on your toes at all times—including while at your resort. In some places, all-inclusive resorts exist because it's poor judgment to wander off the property. How to get and pay for medical treatment is also something you should research and arrange before you plan any trip abroad.

Cyber precautions may include deleting certain data and apps and suspending social media accounts and non-secure email accounts to prevent others from carelessly posting your location or sending you emails with content your destination country might object to. If you are traveling to a country where cyber security is a concern, I strongly recommend consulting an expert. If you do, ask them before using my precautions, such as installing and using a quality Virtual Private Network (VPN) and using an end-to-end encrypted email service to stay in contact with your loved ones at home (SendInc is free and requires each person to have an account; ProtonMail offers their basic encrypted service for free).

If you plan your trip months ahead, get just enough online language practice (I recommend Innovative Language) that you can ask and *be able to listen to* the local language. This shows respect for the culture of your destination country and makes you *much* more welcome—you can't imagine the difference. It is well worth the effort.

The US State Department maintains a list of travel advisories and information about crime abroad, as does the State Department's Overseas Security Advisory Council. Our Centers for Disease Control and Prevention (https://www.cdc.gov/) maintains advice for travelers. You've paid for these resources, so take advantage of them.

* * *

Speaking of world travel, two-time Welsh Olympic Taekwondo champion for Great Britain Jade Jones demonstrates part of her stretching routine in THIS VIDEO[135]

---

[135] "Jade Jones's top tips - Flexibility" (accessed November 10, 2023); available from https://www.youtube.com/watch?v=TCGVveHeObk

14

LEADERSHIP

The person who has confidence in herself
gains the confidence of others. – Hasidic saying (paraphrased)

C arly Fiorina says that a manager does the best she can within an existing situation. Conversely, a leader does not accept things just because they've always been a certain way.

Leadership is a choice and leaders aren't born, they are made when people decide to do something new—something else.

Leadership requires change but people resist this because it can be uncomfortable. Leadership, then, requires courage and being confident enough that you gain others' confidence.

You now have tools your family and friends lack—and may someday need. Using your skills in service of others is called servant leadership. Use your knowledge to keep your group safe. This will require boldness, and practicing the skills in this book will boost your confidence, which makes being bold more natural.

Choose your leader carefully. Sometimes, a leader is the first to recognize a problem or come up with a solution. A leader may be the only person who hasn't given up or has the courage to speak up. Your awareness may equip you to be the first person in your group to recognize a threat or a risky idea—don't keep that a secret.

The highest form of leadership is by example. Set a good, informed example and wise people will follow your lead.

* * *

Check out THIS HIGHLIGHTS REEL[136] of USA men's three-time Olympic Taekwondo medalist, Steven Lopez. This shows the kicks for which Taekwondo is famous. If you decide to commit to long term training and kicking appeals to you, Taekwondo will train you in all kinds of kicks. And because it is an Olympic event, TKD schools are very common.

Regarding the difference between the above-linked international *competition* (with its associated rules and point scoring) and using Taekwondo for *self-protection*: if facing an attacker, low kicks don't require much flexibility and are less likely to leave you open to counterattack during an assault. **High "headhunter" international competition kicks are not used for self-protection**, so don't be concerned if you lack an Olympian's flexibility. Also, in most US TKD studios we train to use our hands nearly as much as our feet.

---

[136] "Taekwondo Legend~Steven Lopez || 3x Olympic Medalist || Best player of USA!" (accessed November 10, 2023); available from: https://www.youtube.com/watch?v=AUDwon4bj-I

15

TRAINING TIPS

"I welcome you to the community of people who have decided that EASY will no longer suffice." —*Mark Rippetoe*[137]

---

[137] https://quotlr.com/author/mark-rippetoe

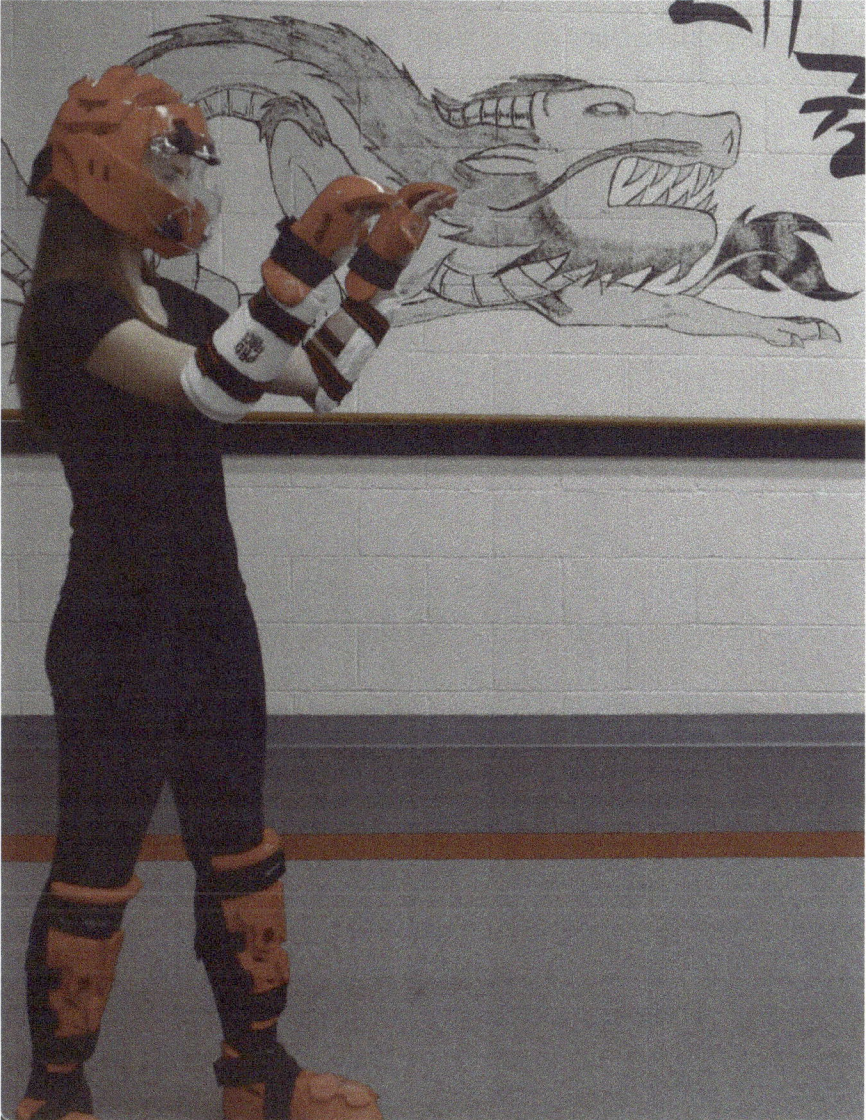

Universal "stay away" command: hands up and shout BACKOFF!

S
elf-defense (fighting back) is hard. *Really* hard. I've had the privilege of training with world- and nationally ranked martial artists as well as law enforcement officers and those who train our law enforcement and counter-terrorism warriors. Nevertheless, I have not met anyone who

claims to be a self-defense expert. Fights are terrifying, violent chaos. That's not a reason to avoid training, that's a reason to train to avoid fighting—*and to know how fight to escape if you need to.*

Seek training that spends significant time focusing on awareness, recognition, de-escalation/avoidance skills and judgment. It helps to role play common attack scenarios to rapidly improve your preparation and confidence, in the same way airlines use simulators to train their pilots in emergency situations. Your goal is to train so you never need to fight. See our Awareness & Avoidance Training Scenarios in the Pulling It All Together chapter.

If you can find a class that uses a padded instructor as police and our Athena Women course use, that is a *big* benefit.

Fighting techniques that you have only memorized over a short time will not be available to you during an assault when your higher thinking ability vanishes. There is no such thing as "one-and-done" training in fighting back anymore than a few lessons without follow-up practice will make you proficient at playing tennis or guitar. **Practice until executing your techniques feels as natural as your startle reaction.** Note the difference between "I suppose (*sigh*) I should probably sign up for a self-defense class" and "I am going to train to be able to protect myself."

The number of repetitions required for competence varies greatly from person to person, and not all repetitions are equally helpful. Not surprisingly, the more alive (realistic) you can make your repetitions, the swifter your progress. Practicing with a resisting, moving training partner or padded instructor is superior to striking a bag, which is superior to hitting air. Practice or train at least two to three times per week, alternating what skills you hone. Do this and you *will* improve faster than you can imagine.

Tip for success:

Adding practice time to your day's routine requires first deciding what you will do less of, or reschedule, in order to free up training time.

What Should My Training Look Like?

Fighting skills are often divided into two groups: *striking* (mostly fighting on your feet using hands, feet, elbows, and knees) and *grappling* (grabs, joint locks, chokes, wrestling). Almost all schools now incorporate both types of skills to some degree. Some striking techniques are also used while on the ground, and some grappling moves are useful while standing.

A well-thought-out short course in fighting back will *not* consist of complicated, multi-step techniques. Nevertheless, the course will probably reflect the school's main interest—striking or grappling. Look for a course that teaches *striking* skills aimed at providing opportunities to run away, as well as *escapes* from being restrained both on your feet and on the ground. Because demand for short-term training is thin, you probably won't have much if any choice.

If you cannot find local training or you want to augment your in-studio training, there is of course online training. If you decide to learn online I strongly suggest getting some basic fighting training to learn primary fighting movements and concepts, both to get your technique correct and to avoid injuries. Not everything online is worth your time but there are some high spots. Here are sources I recommend that focus on various skills (as always, take what you find useful, discard what you do not):

- Code Red Defense™ videos by Nick Drossos and Patrick Viana. [138] Drossos worked the door at clubs (AKA bouncer) for seven years and has ring fighting experience. Everything he shows is real-world, pressure-tested self-protection tactics and techniques, including defending against weapons. This is mostly striking—because that is where most fights begin and where you have the best chance of escaping unharmed. No uniforms, no flashy but unrealistic movements from action movies, Code Red Defense is messy and chaotic like real life. Caution for some rough language. Get their Awareness video. They have many short videos online that you can take a lot away from, plus longer videos for sale. Much of it is aimed at male vs. male fighting, but you will learn something from each

---

[138] https://www.coderreddefense.com

of their videos. Your understanding of how to deal with predators and real life fighting will *greatly* expand from watching these videos. This training is about **dealing with attackers from start to finish with the goal of preventing a confrontation from becoming physical, and escaping unharmed if it does**. If you are beginning, I suggest you start here to get the big picture.

- Gracie Breakdown videos (women's self defense series) by the innovative, world-champion Gracie Jiu Jitsu family. [139] This focuses on self protection concepts and especially very effective, proven grappling escapes from realistic assault situations. **These ground skills are crucial, _especially for women._** This is a top-shelf organization.
- Krav Maga Training (Italy) [140] Krav Maga ("contact combat") is strictly for self-protection; it originated with the Israeli Defense Forces for short-term training. Krav Maga teaches natural, gross muscle movements. It uses striking and grappling techniques. **Krav Maga is a well-rounded fighting system** taught worldwide; I chose this Italian school because they have posted many videos (with English subtitles). The name Krav Maga is not trademarked, anyone can open a school and use the name. The way to know whether a school is certified by the worldwide organization is to look for the trademarked KM logo (that this school does use, along with its own).

Here are three metrics to think about during your local or online shopping:

- Focused self-protection training should focus on *head work*: awareness, predator habits, and knowing, recognizing, and avoiding common attacks and then practicing countering those scenarios.
- Fighting techniques shown to you must be *simple* to do using only *gross motor skills*, and consist of a *minimum number of movements* that make sense to you.
- The tactics and techniques must work against a *moving, reacting* attacker.

---

[139] https://www.youtube.com/playlist?list=PLl1zLMTQrUzhvPs-AzqpeO-db5K_Dh6P2

[140] https://www.kravmagatraining.it/en/videos/

As a general rule, deliberately taking an attacker down to the ground is risky. He may have an unseen nearby accomplice or a weapon—either of which could be *fatal* to you while you're more vulnerable on the ground. Additionally, staying on your feet may more quickly provide an opportunity to flee. For those reasons, I do not recommend prioritizing your training on taking down attackers to "finish the fight". That said, it is a good idea (and fun) to be skilled at both escaping from being held down *and* escaping on your feet.

Some physical fighting concepts you should learn during training that help take away some of the advantages a larger, stronger attacker has are:

- *Surprise!*
- Unbalancing the attacker
- Maintaining your own balance with a strong stance
- Protecting yourself—especially your head using cover-up blocking—then switching from defense to offense as soon as you can ("defensive offense")
- Controlling distance: being out of his striking range when you can, closing only when you need to be to facilitate fighting back by striking or grappling
- Focusing your body's mass and strength on a smaller, vulnerable part of the attacker's body

The following photos are presented only to give you an idea of striking vs. grappling and the kinds of simple escapes you might learn in a short-term training program. These pictures do not teach you how to perform these techniques. None of these techniques is shown in its entirety. For those of you who'd like to learn fighting from a book, an instructional book on fighting from this author will depend on how enthusiastically this book is received. To avoid injury, do NOT try to perform these or any other fighting movements without medical clearance, professional instruction, and full martial arts protective equipment for both training partners.

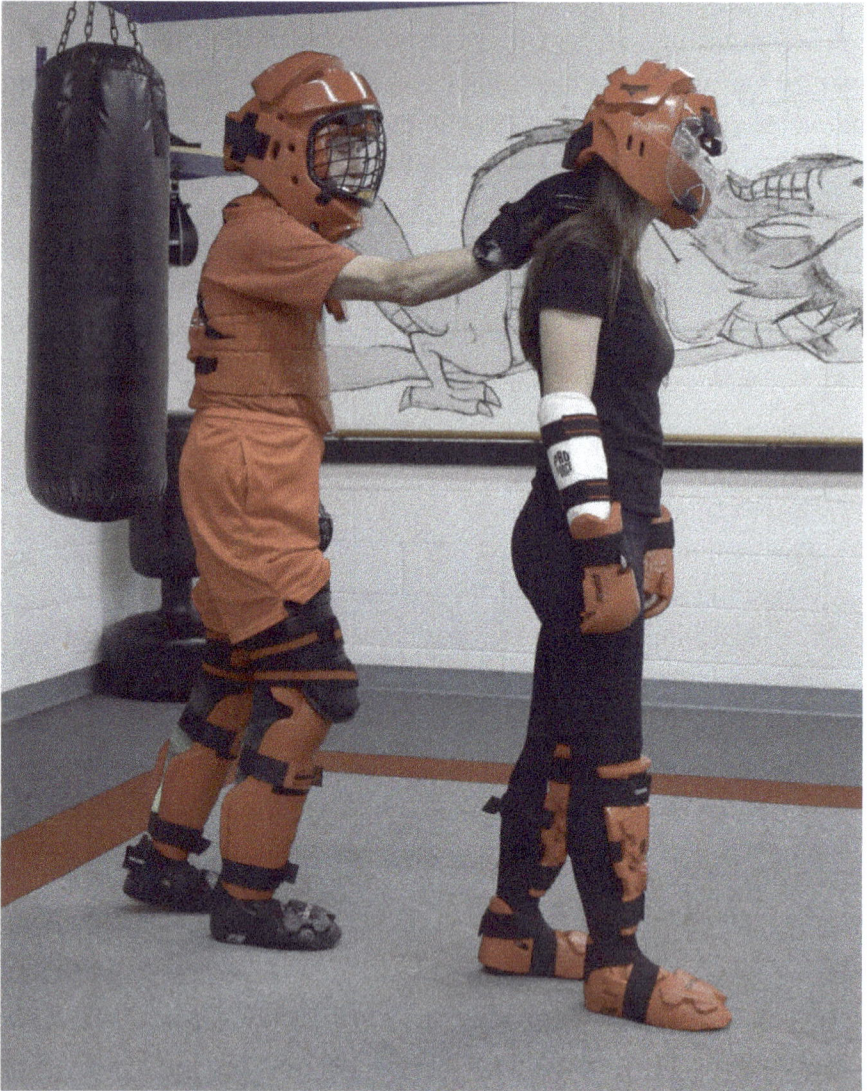

Attacker grabs defender's hair or clothing from behind.

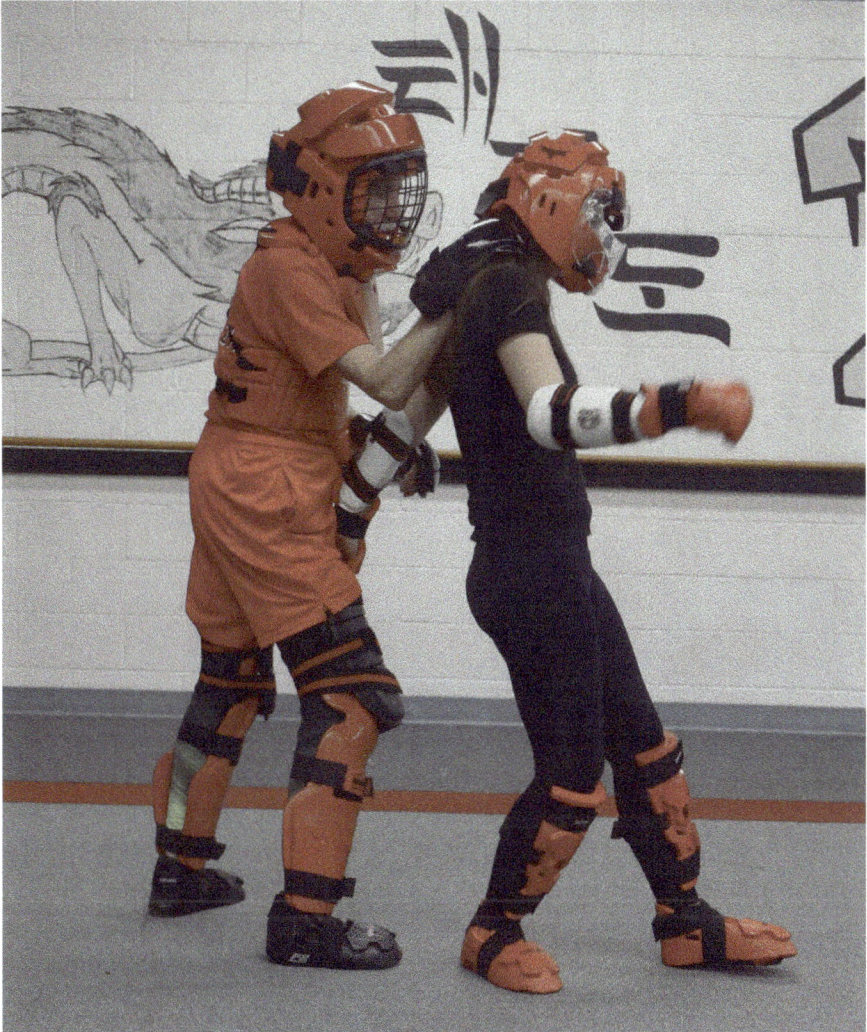

Surprise: Defender lunges backward into attacker and counterattacks to put him on defense so she can turn around and fight back.

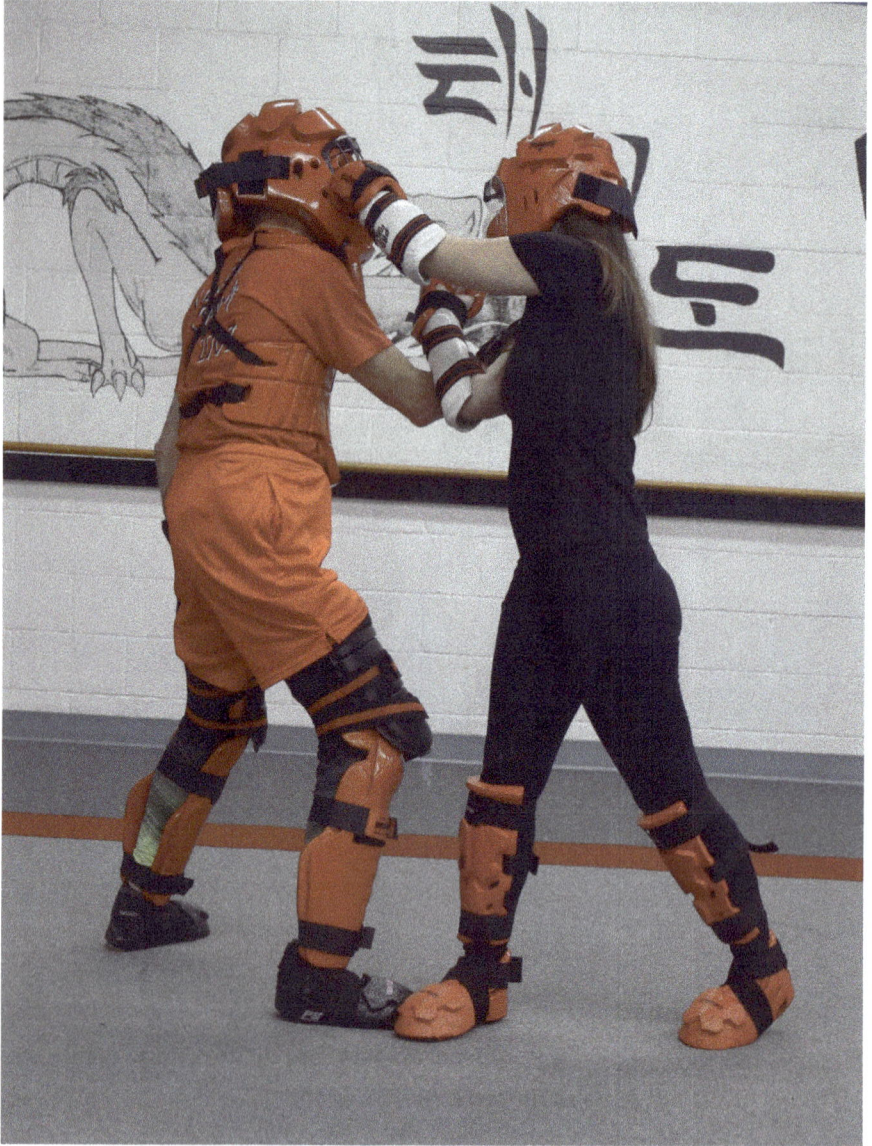

Defender counterattacks until she has an opportunity to flee.

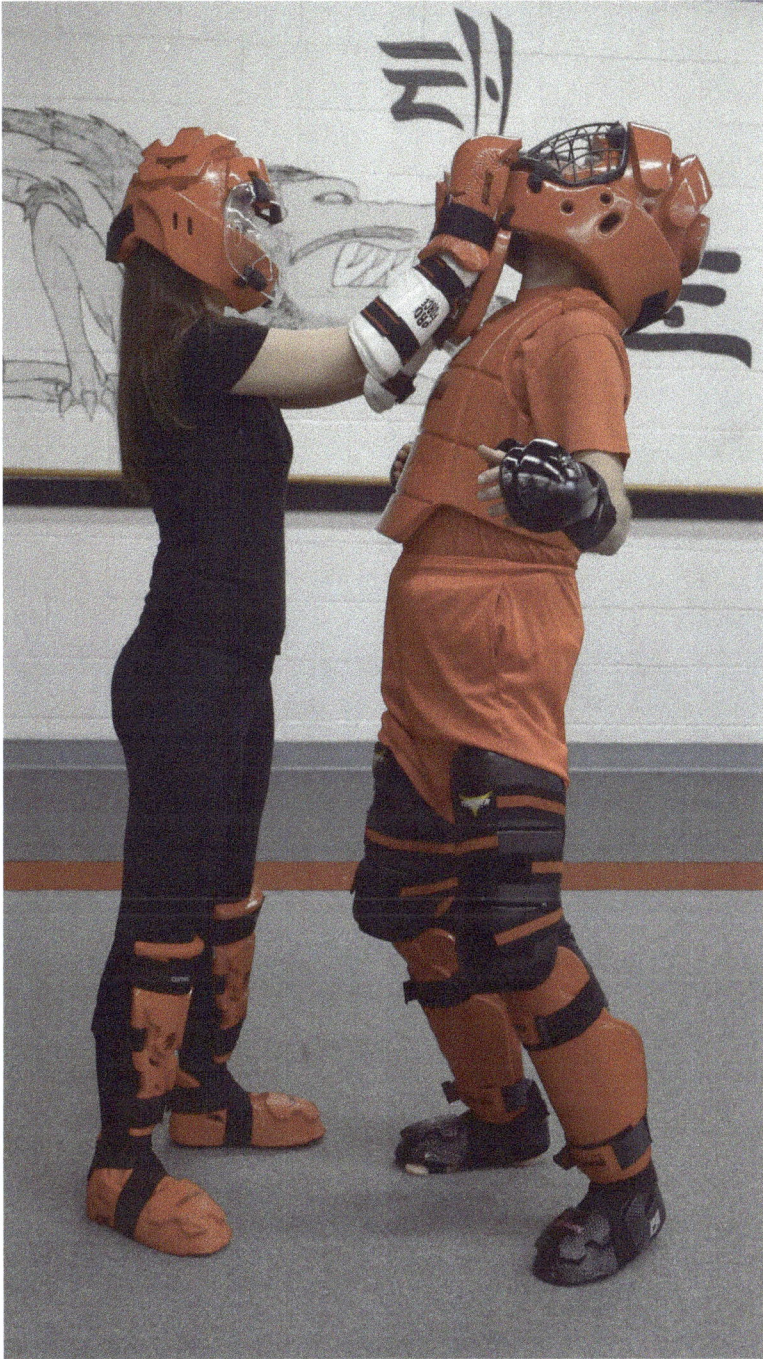

A double palm strike can be a powerful blow.

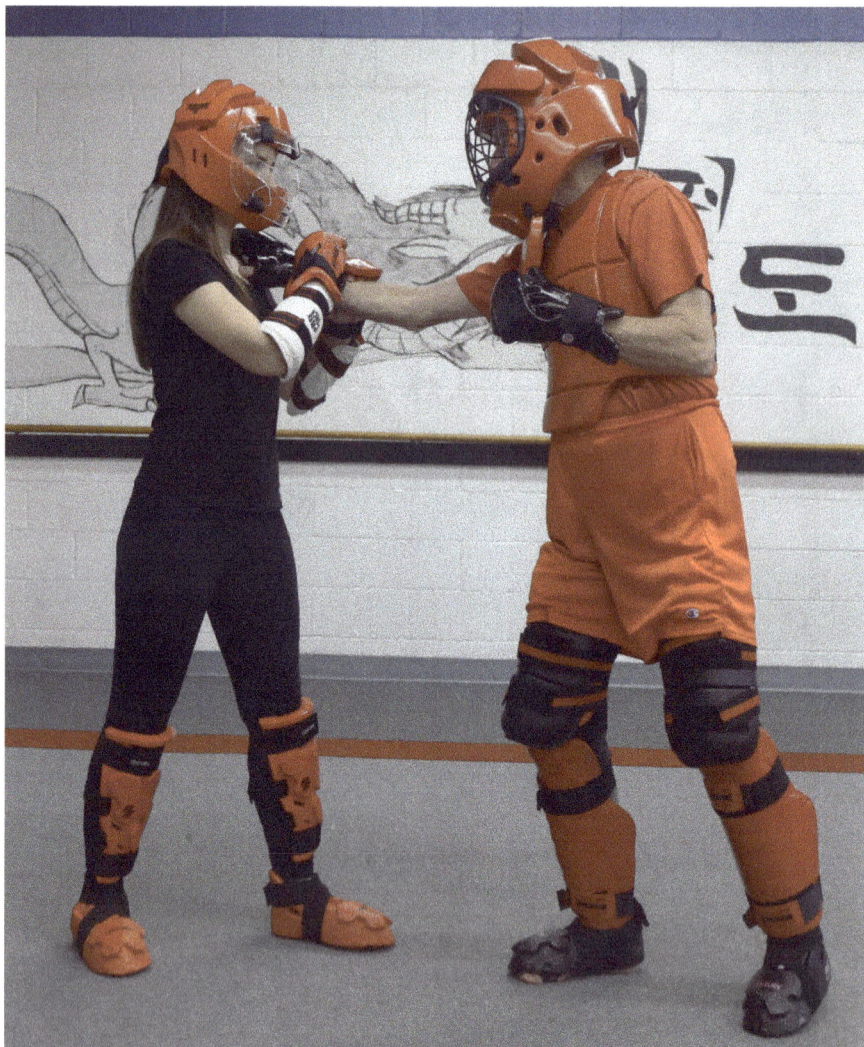

Assailant grabs throat or collar with one hand; defender will lift her right elbow to guard her head against getting punched and to begin the escape.

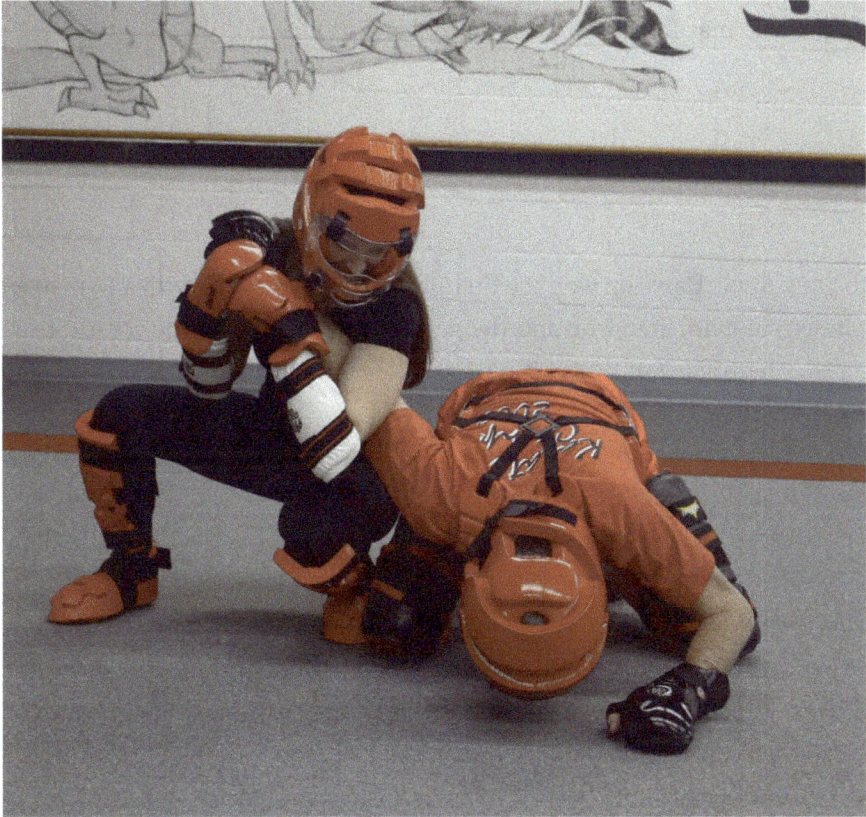

Defender will end this technique in a way that allows her to flee safely. Photos: Gail Lewis

Tip for success:

Choose the art and school that you think you will appreciate spending time with so you will look forward to classes and want to practice. Here's a video[141] about practicing without a partner.

For me, the consequences of not being prepared to repel a violent predator are unacceptable and outweigh the effort and time spent to prepare. Your risk analysis rests with you, and you deserve to thoughtfully settle this decision.

---

[141] "How to Practice Martial Arts Alone – Solo Training Tip" (accessed November 10, 2023); available from https://www.youtube.com/watch?v=1jYk9JWwgl4

Bonus: you may fall in love with martial arts as I have.

* * *

In 2012, Kayla Harrison won the first Olympic Gold Medal for the US (men or women) in judo, then won another gold in 2016. She currently competes in MMA, where she is at this writing 8-0.

Her struggle to personal victory is even more impressive. Check out her Fearless Foundation[142].

WATCH THIS[143] video of Harrison's first Olympic Gold Medal finals match as an introduction to a grappling art. Relax: competition judo's powerful throws—suitable mostly for younger people—are *not* among skills needed to escape an attacker or taught in short-term training.

---

[142] Kayla Harrison's Olympic final match: https://www.youtube.com/watch?v=7B4yzmf6FEQ

[143] "Kayla Harrison Wins Women's Judo -78kg Gold v Gemma Gibbons - London 2012 Olympics" (accessed November 10, 2023); available from https://www.youtube.com/watch?v=7B4yzmf6FEQ

16

STAYING SAFE DURING TRAINING

"The less effort, the faster and more powerful you will be." —*Bruce Lee*

- The first goal is for everyone to go home able to perform normal activities and return to train the following session. Getting hurt is no fun and injured students can't train.

- Pain is your body warning you to cease what you're doing. PAIN = STOP.

- Work within your body's limits. Do not attempt any technique—or allow any technique to be practiced on you—that you suspect may exceed your range of motion or otherwise cause you pain or injury.

- If you are not comfortable performing a technique, ask for help.

- If while doing repetitions you begin to notice soreness creeping in, it is past time to cease training or work with a different part of your body.

- Performing techniques incorrectly can lead to injury. If instructions aren't clear to you, ask.

- Tell your instructor if you have an existing injury so that she or he can help you avoid making it worse.

- Before class begins, tell your instructor if you have medication you might need someone to help you with during class, such as an inhaler.

- If you need water or a break, take it.

- If you are experiencing pain or think you may be injured, or feel light-headed or short of breath, immediately stop training and tell an instructor.

- If you see anyone else appearing to be in distress, tell an instructor.

- A common error you must avoid is demanding too much of yourself too soon by trying to perform intensely instead of correctly. This is a prelude to injury. Focus on *correct execution of technique* and the speed and power will naturally come to you with practice. Focus on speed and power and you will not achieve technique good enough to protect you.

- If you need to stop or see an unsafe situation, yell out the safe word: "Break!"

- Stay relaxed and have fun!

Joe Rogan says you train so you won't have to worry.
You want to be the one who gets to decide how to handle the other person.

* * *

You've seen striking in the Steven Lopez Olympic Taekwondo highlight reel at the end of the Leadership chapter, and grappling in Kayla Harrison's Olympic gold medal judo match at the end of the Training Tips chapter.

IF YOU WATCH ONLY ONE VIDEO FROM THIS BOOK, MAKE IT THIS ONE:
THIS VIDEO[144] puts striking and a bit of grappling together in simple self-

---

[144] Chuck Norris Teaches Self-Defense (accessed November 10, 2023); available from https://www.dailymotion.com/video/x4bi250

defense techniques. Chuck Norris narrates this demonstration of a well-trained woman fighting off a large, male assailant in a few different types of attacks. Most of the techniques shown can be learned and used by people who have no previous fighting training.

17

PARENTS & GUARDIANS

"As with anything in life, you have to wait for the game to come to you." —*Dennis Miller*

We ask that you invest time going over this book with your daughter. Avoidance is the first step in not getting attacked and it is the point of this material.

This training is necessary, in part, to give your youth permission to break out of the polite social conventions you've worked so hard to instill within them. Of course this book is not aimed at dealing with polite people who respect your child.

Once a physical attack is underway, there is no such thing as a fair fight. People with evil intentions have already decided that getting what they want is more important than the law, their victim's wellness, dignity, or even her life.

During Athena Women classes, we encourage appropriate techniques as well as verbal commands. As each lesson progresses, we increase the intensity of the training so as to elevate your youth's adrenaline level. We want her to feel what it will be like to fight under stress. You may see her react with ferocity you've never imagined.

Please do not critique or discourage this intensity. Your approval and support of your daughter is necessary for her to internalize this training.

We respect you as the parent and ultimate authority. We're honored that you've chosen to trust us to train your daughter. We're confident you will be pleased with the end result.

18

RESOURCES

(I receive no compensation from any of the companies mentioned in this book.)

Training in the Korean arts of Tae Kwon Do, Tang Soo Do, Hap Ki Do, American Tal Chul Do, and various weapons: Kreimer's Karate Institute

"Your Happy Little Dragon," by this author, in the February/March 2015 issue of *Frederick's Child* magazine (pp 20-23; available printed or online at http://www.mydigitalpublication.com/publication/?i=242370). Valid for adults, too.

Code Red Defense™ realistic self-protection videos. Caution for some rough language.

Gracie Breakdown women's self-protection videos, as well as other self-defense series.

Krav Maga Training (Italy, subtitles). Focused self-protection.

Westview Psychological Counseling Service

Ayoob, Massad, *The Truth About Self Protection* (Concord: Police Bookshelf, 1999)

RAINN: Rape, Abuse & Incest National Network: https://rainn.org/

Maryland sex offenders: https://www.dpscs.state.md.us/onlineservs/socem/default.shtml

Sun Tzu, *Sun Tzu on the Art Of War.* The 1910 translation by Lionel Giles is in the public domain. http://www.au.af.mil/au/awc/awcgate/artofwar.htm or downloaded at
   http://www.loyalbooks.com/book/the-art-of-war-by-sun-tzu

Is someone lying to you? "Former CIA Officers Share 6 Ways to Tell If Someone's Lying" *Parade*, July 25, 2013. Accessed December 18, 2015. http://parade.com/57236/vianguyen/former-cia-officers-share-6-ways-to-tell-if-someones-lying/

Cyber Security: "Internet Privacy Evangelist," Rob Braxman (https://brax.me/home/rob)
   Plain language online safety website: (https://staysafeonline.org/stay-safe-online/)
   "Once Posted, You Lose It." (https://www.youtube.com/watch?v=CE2Ru-jqyrY)
   Social network privacy loss: (https://www.youtube.com/watch?v=-e98hxHZiTg)
   Internet Safety For Teens: (https://www.youtube.com/watch?t=60&v=QoPe-skp4Nc)
   To see how VPNs work, watch this short video: https://www.youtube.com/watch?v=SuD7aZQ4aq4
   Data Google has amassed on you: (https://accounts.google.com/signin/v2/identifier?passive=1209600&osid=1&continue=https%3A%2F%2Ftakeout.google.com%2Fsettings%2Ftakeout&followup=https%3A%2F%2Ftakeo

ut.google.com%2Fsettings%2Ftakeout&flowName=GlifWebSignIn&flowEn try=ServiceLogin)

To see your data Facebook has scooped up: (https://www.facebook.com/ help/131112897028467)

Online tracking: (https://robertheaton.com/2017/11/20/how-does-online -tracking-actually-work/)

Facebook incident timeline: (https://www.creativefuture.org/facebook- scandal-timeline/)

19

TWO RULES FOR SUCCESS!

"THERE ARE TWO RULES FOR BEING SUCCESSFUL IN MARTIAL ARTS.

RULE 1: NEVER TELL OTHERS EVERYTHING YOU KNOW."

— unknown

And HERE [145] is that advice in (humorous) action!

---

[145] "Fighter Surprises Pros With Kickboxing and MMA Moves" (accessed November 10, 2023); available from https://www.youtube.com/watch?v=F3FZLTpJREY

20

ATHENA WOMEN SELF-PROTECTION CHEAT SHEET

(Print & Post!)

Some common Threats:

- **"All warfare is deception." Predators are skilled at not raising your suspicion.**
- Higher threat places: parking and commercial areas, schools, residences
- Distraction: Predator approaches victim, who he engages in conversation (sucker punch attack with one or more assailants); often in parking areas or on streets
- **Triple-A** attacks: you're **A**lone, or not paying **A**ttention, or when **A**lcohol is consumed
- **Double-I** (**I**ntoxicate & **I**solate) attack.
- Tackle from behind on exercise path (sexual assault)
- Sexual assault in residences, especially by known, drinking males
- Entering or exiting our cars, including at home
- Unlocking the doors to enter your home or responding to a knock at the door

- Sexual attacks can begin close to you and slowly.
- Habits and routines are powerful and can override your survival instinct.
- Violent attacks happen sooner, closer, faster and more viciously than you think.
- His strikes will injure you more than you expect, and yours will damage him less than you expect.
- **Complacency kills.**

Countermeasures to help you avoid or mitigate the above situations:

- Keep your head on a swivel & frequently "check six".
- Listen to your gut when it tells you something's wrong.
- Think of risk in terms of consequences, not merely probability.
- If his body language disagrees with his mouth language, believe his body.
- Run—not walk—away from anyone who is trying to pour alcohol down your throat, separate you from your friends, gain your personal information, or doesn't take "no" for an answer.
- Guard your personal information, especially online.
- Everyone is *not* "just like me"; make *everyone* earn your trust over time.
- Rude Is the New Safe (your safety trumps others' feelings).
- Project the image of a Hard Target: alert, confident, but not challenging.
- *Different* is a Red Flag.
- Know two safe directions in which you might flee.
- Establish and defend your bubble verbally—and physically if needed.
- "Back off!" is a command and the *last* line in a conversation.
- Aware—Avoid/De-escalate—Flee—Comply—(Counter)attack (5 Step Plan)
- "Complying" refers to robberies and does *not* include surrendering to a sexual assault and *never* includes going to the deadly second crime scene.
- You survive an attack by going and staying on offense: learn to fight back.
- If you cannot positively determine that a Threat's hands are empty, assume he is armed. (*Watch hands. Hands kill.*)

· A physical attack can maim or kill you so do not physically engage a Threat unless there is no alternative. This warning times 10 if he is armed.

21

ABOUT THE AUTHOR AND ATHENA WOMEN SELF-PROTECTION CREATOR

S cott Lewis's 34-year career as a professional pilot began as most civilian piloting careers do: flight instructing. He taught at the Florida Institute of Technology School of Aeronautics and discovered a passion for teaching. While he never outright taught at airlines, 21 of the 29 years he flew for a major airline were as captain, which is a mentoring position. Scott applied modern flight training methods to the material in this book and his in-studio instruction.

Scott, a fifth-degree black belt, believes that smaller, less-robust people have a right to confidently and proactively protect themselves. In addition to women's self-protection, he has taught traditional martial arts classes in Korean Karate that combines Tae Kwon Do, Tang Soo Do and Hap Ki Do as well as weapons at Kreimer's Karate Institute. Scott co-developed and co-teaches with two other instructors at Kreimer's Karate a street fighting syllabus, Tal Chul Do (way of escape), which incorporates some Athena Women training.

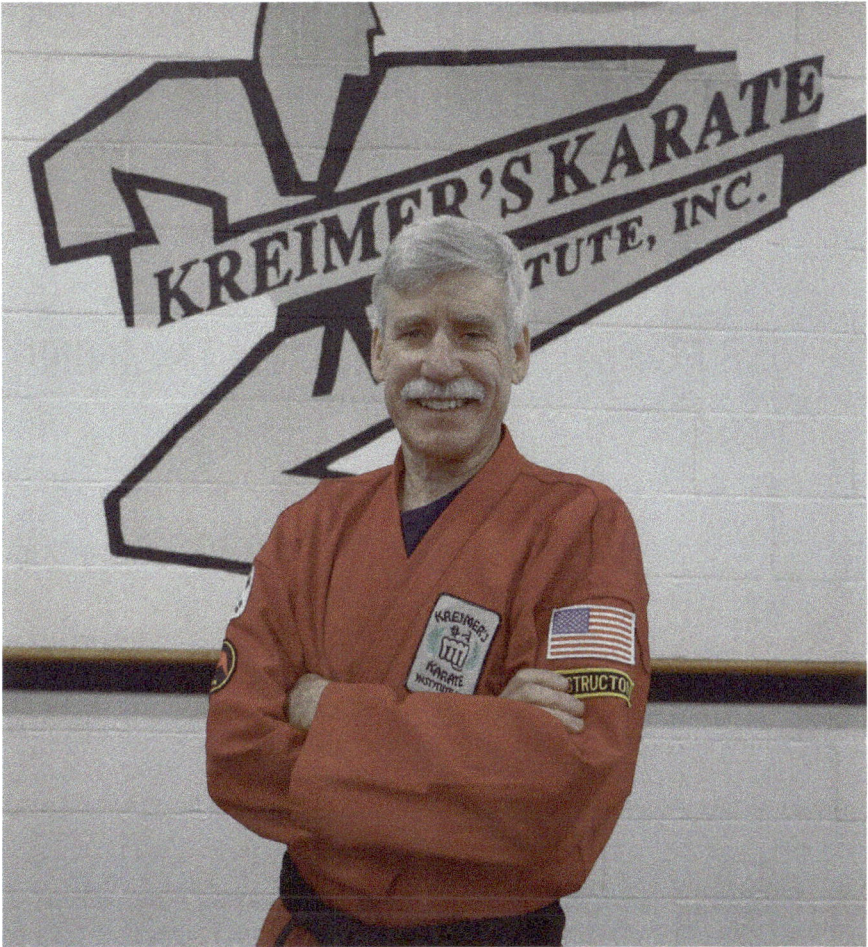

Other works by Scott Lewis:

"Your Happy Little Dragon", *Frederick's Child* magazine (https://cdn.coversta
nd.com/6734/242370/2923d4b6d567bb4166bfdcb0cf89dad7c3c56a22.5.pdf)

"Airplane Self-Defenselessness", WND.com

(https://www.wnd.com/2002/02/12898)

22

PRAISE FOR ATHENA WOMEN TRAINING

"We signed up our 14-year-old daughter G. with instructor Scott in the Athena Women's defense tactics class.

"Great class, 2-hour blocks of instruction, Scott taught situational awareness, tactics and instilled confidence. We highly recommend this class to any young lady. The tactics were current and relative to everyday situations. Many thanks to instructor Scott and Kreimer's Karate.

"Respectfully,

M.B and J.H." —Law Enforcement Officer

* * *

"...your program and your passion about it had and still has such a positive impact on my life." —student K.U.

* * *

"I really have seen the great effects of even thinking about self defense/safety frequently." —student A.H.

* * *

"I appreciate you still looking out for your students. That means a lot."
—student E.D.

* * *

"Lewis interactively demonstrated common attacks and the venues that
facilitate them, as well as effective countermeasures to violent crimes." —Bill
Anderson, Rotary Club of Fredericktowne as quoted in the *Frederick News-Post,*
April 30, 2019.

* * *

"If you are a local lady this is a great idea. The instructors are great! You will
learn a lot." —Black Belt martial artist A.B.

* * *

"Thank you so much for all you taught me. You are an excellent teacher and
you've helped many people and made the world a better place for women. I
really enjoyed the classes. Good luck to you!" —student B.V.